"When a caregiver wonders *where do I begin*, this book is the answer. Important resource for the caregiver. Good *get down to basics* help."

  Beverly J. Bach, Partner, Shoun, Bach, Walinsky, & Curran, P.C. (Retired)
  Former Director, Fairfax County (VA) Bar Association Board

"The author kept his wife at home longer than any family I can think of. The *matter of fact* style of the book is very compelling. I find it difficult to put it down. This book will serve as a very useful handbook for caregivers that they can keep referring to as they care for their loved one with a progressive dementing illness. It will serve a real need for a practical *nuts and bolts* approach to caregiving. This book is loaded with practical tips."

  Andrew A. Schiavone, M.D.
  Former Assistant Clinical Professor, Georgetown University Medical School
  Multiple selections as one of the Woodward and White's *Best Doctors in America*

"This is a unique book. It describes in useful and personal detail the experiences learned. Few, if any, others have documented their experiences, their procedures, personal feelings, successes and failures as is done in this volume. Frank's report and guidance born of experience can be a huge benefit. This ready reference to successful caregiving should be in every home faced with a dementia case, and perhaps those caring for other chronically ill loved ones. Use of Frank's advice can save countless hours of painful experimentation and enable more time to enjoy the quality of life that may remain with each patient."

  Rear Admiral Donald M. Showers, USN (Retired), longtime caregiver and former
  Director, Alzheimer's Association, National Capitol Area Chapter Board

"In reviewing Frank's account of his wife's battle with Alzheimer's disease, it is impossible not to be moved by his obvious love and compassion. He has shared with us the many difficult lessons he has learned as her caregiver to benefit others in a similar situation. We are all enriched by his dignity and courage."

  Joanne G. Crantz, M.D.
  Division Chief, Geriatrics, Inova Fairfax Hospital
  Assistant Professor of Medicine, George Washington University

"What Frank has written is accurate and factual. Well done!"

  Bruce W. Jay, D.D.S., P.C.
  Former Assistant Professor of Dentistry, Georgetown University

"Frank has done an excellent job of researching the subject and compiling his thoughts. These are helpful suggestions for all situations regarding terminal illnesses. He has done a fine job of presenting the necessary steps and issues when dealing with this disease."

  Marvin G. Parker, M.D., FACP
  VP Corporate Medical Affairs, SC Johnson (Retired).

"The accurate technical information is important and Frank does an excellent job. What is more important is that those reading Frank's book will know that they are not alone. Caregiving can be a lonely job and many view their exhaustion, loneliness and frustration as unique. While each specific situation may be unique, it is crucial for caregivers to feel connected, to understand that it is common to feel angry, impatient, and frustrated. I commend Frank for sharing not only information, but emotions as well."

  Jane Marks, Executive Director
  Alzheimer's Association, West Virginia Chapter

Alzheimer's Care with Dignity

by
Frank Fuerst

To order additional copies of the book,
see order form after the Index

Limited First Edition

Contact the author:

Frank Fuerst
carewithdignity@earthlink.net
www.dementiacaregiving.com

ISBN 0929915623

Library of Congress Control Number: 2007925751

Alzheimer's care with dignity: a handbook of solutions for caring for someone with dementia at home from diagnosis through final stages.
Includes index.
Includes bibliography.
1. Alzheimer's. 2. Caregiving. 3. Dementia. 4. Long-term care. 5. Self-care, Health.

Front Cover Photo by Takahase Segundo , Brazil
Back Cover Photo by Clifton Grim,USA

PRINTED IN THE UNITED STATES OF AMERICA

Alzheimer's Care with Dignity

by
Frank Fuerst

Copyrights and Permissions

Disclaimers

Any mention of a particular product or supplier does not imply an
endorsement of that product or supplier. These products and suppliers are merely
a starting point to enable a caregiver to do a comparative analysis with other
products and suppliers.

Neither the author nor the publisher is engaged in tendering medical,
legal, accounting, or other professional advice. If one requires such advice or
other assistance, one should seek the services of a competent professional.

"There aren't any great men. There are just great challenges that ordinary men are forced by circumstances to meet."
Fleet Admiral William F. (Bull) Halsey, Jr., U.S. Navy, at Guadalcanal World War II
(from *The Gallant Hours)*

This book is dedicated to all of the caregivers who are meeting the great challenges

and to the memory of my late wife,

June

and to the memory of my late son,

Jeff

Table of Contents

Preface 9

Acknowledgments 11

Not in a Sliver Casket with Pearls 12

Prologue 13

CHAPTER 1   SECRETS OF SURVIVAL 15

CHAPTER 2   OUR SEVENTEEN YEARS 27

CHAPTER 3   FINANCIAL CONCERNS 40

CHAPTER 4   LEGAL CONCERNS 48

CHAPTER 5   DENTAL 51

CHAPTER 6   MEDICAL 55

CHAPTER 7   PRESCRIPTION DRUGS 63

CHAPTER 8   PRODUCTS THAT WORK 69

CHAPTER 9   WHEN OTHERS PROVIDE CARE 88

CHAPTER 10   OTHER RESOURCES 108

DAY BY DAY LIVING

CHAPTER 11   BATHING 116

CHAPTER 12 DRESSING/UNDRESSING 121

CHAPTER 13 EATING 126

CHAPTER 14 CONTINENCE AND INCONTINENCE 134

CHAPTER 15 MOVING FROM PLACE TO PLACE 137

CHAPTER 16 OTHER TIPS 149

CHAPTER 17 GOOD EXAMPLES OF BAD ADVICE 176

EPILOGUE 180

APPENDIX A MUSIC VIDEOS 181
APPENDIX B ACTIVITIES OF DAILY LIVING 182
APPENDIX C FOOD RECIPES 183
APPENDIX D MENTAL STATUS TESTS 184
APPENDIX E SAMPLES OF NIH STUDIES 185
APPENDIX F EMERGENCY MEDICAL DATA 187
APPENDIX G HELPFUL CARE HINTS 188
APPENDIX H LIVE-IN AGREEMENT (SAMPLE) 190
APPENDIX I CLOTHING INVENTORY 191
APPENDIX J PERCENT OF RESPITE COST 192
APPENDIX K VOCABULARY 193
APPENDIX L MAINTAINING SKILLS 194
BIBLIOGRAPHY 195
INDEX 201

Preface

After doctors diagnosed June Fuerst with early onset Alzheimer's disease (AD), her husband attended lectures and read every available book and article on the subject. He followed most advice and found what worked, and what did not. He kept daily notes. As the disease progressed, he found himself in uncharted territory and relied on his own creativity and a process of trial and error. He realized that some information he needed was not available from any source.

In June 2006, the Alzheimer's Association confirmed his realization. They focused attention on the early onset of AD to a Congressional task force. Their report said, "When they occur in people under age 65, the conditions [dementia] cause additional and unique problems because they are so unexpected and because most of the potentially helpful programs and services are designed for and targeted to older people." They went on to cover six major problems confronted by people with early onset dementia and their families. The sixth problem was especially significant. "Doctors and other . . . providers may not know how to treat, provide care for, or communicate with people with early onset dementia. Training to address this problem is not generally available, and much of the information that would be needed as a basis for such training does not exist."

This book supplies much of that information. It contains practical solutions to the six problems stated by the Alzheimer's Association and all of the other challenges faced by those caring for a family member. Its completeness reflects the author's first hand experience of seventeen years. It discusses many helpful products and resources. It presents ways of solving problems of behavior, communications, prescription drugs, emotions, mobility, personal care, and safety. Its tailored advice includes solutions to problems that can arise when dealing with finances, dentists, doctors, lawyers, and part-time caregivers. These solutions are effective, simple, inexpensive, clear, and concise. Alphabetical topics within chapters make reference easy. Universal solutions will also help with other incapacitating illnesses. Organizations could use it as a basis for training, and caregivers can now get the help they need.

Caregivers desperately look to long-term care insurance and government subsidized nursing homes as solutions. Unfortunately, long-term care insurance is still an unproven solution. It is currently in its collecting phase, and has yet to make substantial payments. Many policies contain a provision that grants the insurance company the right to apply to state insurance commissions for across-the-board increases based on total claims. The May 2004 AARP Bulletin cited a case of a 61% increase in rates over a two-year period.

In addition, government bodies now realize they cannot fund the tidal wave of needs that many people will generate. The federal government has already decreased Medicaid matching grants to states. To solve their budget crises, all states have reduced or frozen Medicaid provider payments. To control drug costs, they now require prior authorization and preferred drug lists. Two-thirds of the states have also reduced or restricted eligibility, reduced benefits, and increased co-payments.

With budgets shrinking and needs rising, a shift of government subsidies toward home care would be more cost-effective. Most caregivers would prefer this, but may not have enough knowledge to be effective. The solutions in this book allowed the author to care for his wife for the entire length of her illness. Health care professionals acknowledged his unique situation by telling him that he kept his wife at home longer than any other Alzheimer's patient they knew.

This book omits information that is readily available. For example, in the first chapter, the definition of and the justification for negative emotions gives way to the resolution of this behavior. Likewise, voluminous and rapidly obsolete research data is missing, but the reader learns how to get the most current data. Thus, the solutions that are included pick up where others leave off. These solutions show how to care for suffering family members while maintaining their dignity.. They also tell how to protect a caregiver's own health.

Acknowledgments

Although an army seemed to support me, special thanks go to the following:

My son Frank, his wife Karen, their daughters Marissa and Adrienne, my daughter Kathy, her sons Bryan, Evan, and Nicholas, and my mother-in-law Louise Parker. They stuck with me throughout June's illness, encouraged me after her death, and reviewed the entire manuscript. My late sister, Margaret Mullenfeld, and my late brother, Gus, and his wife, Maxine, were always there for me.

Our longtime friends, especially Nila Augsburger, Ellen Heitz, Sue and Hank Leopold, Ray Mooney, Rolf Taubner, Ingrid Ward, and Al and Jewell West.

Our McLean and Regency Racquet Club friends, especially Dot and Lou DeWilde, Phyllis and Gary Edwards, Ken and Sharon Kincel, Bill and Miriam Kuhn, Al and Penny Linch, Tonya Nichols, Doris and Jack O'Grady, Bill and Jan Rae, Mary and Woody Taylor, and Charlie and Maggie Van Winkle. They were my early supporters and gave encouragement when I needed it.

My good friends in IBM encouraged me, especially Jack Butler, Susan Cowart, Molly Reed, and Nancy and Paul Weikert. Barth Brooker and his wife Isabel were the first to volunteer as reviewers.

Friends in Harpers Ferry, especially Al and Allison Alsdorf, Deborah and Zan Fleming, and Dorlyn and Bob Williams.

Many others graciously consented to be reviewers, especially Sharon Albert, Beverly Bach, LD, Joanne Crantz, MD, Rev. Georgia DuBose, Bruce Jay, DDS, Janet Kulesh, Marvin Parker, MD, and Andrew Schiavone, MD. Julianne and Boyd Griffin also shared their publishing wisdom.

The Martinsburg Library writers' group gave helpful critiques, especially Joe McCabe, Sally Brinkman, Beverly Rees, and Craig Tucker.

The West Virginia Writers' group gave encouragement and recognition, especially Susan Bedwell, Bonnie Brechbill, and Cat Pleska.

The Alzheimer's Association, especially Mac Showers from the National Capitol Area Chapter, and Jane Marks, Executive Director, West Virginia Chapter.

Not in a Silver Casket Cool with Pearls

Not in a silver casket cool with pearls
Or rich with red corundum or with blue,
Locked, and the key withheld, as other girls
Have given their loves, I give my love to you;
Not in a lovers'-knot, not in a ring
Worked in such fashion, and the legend plain -
Semper fidelis, where a secret spring
Kennels a drop of mischief for the brain:
Love in the open hand, no thing but that,
Ungemmed, unhidden, wishing not to hurt,
As one should bring you cowslips in a hat
Swung from the hand, or apples in her skirt,
I bring you, calling out as children do:
"Look what I have!—And these are all for you."

Edna St. Vincent Millay

Prologue

"Love in the open hand, no thing but that . . ."

The great cruelty of Alzheimer's disease, for the caregiver who must observe and cope with the changes, is the contrast between present realities and bright memories. It was thus with my wife. June was intelligent, articulate, gracious, enthusiastic, vivacious, and had a great sense of humor. She painted landscapes and still life, and loved to travel and eat out. Moves to eleven different cities and other hurdles of life, she took in stride. She had a remarkable combination of charm, gentleness, poise, and manners. Her style and endearing qualities shone in the poem she gave me on our tenth wedding anniversary, *Not in a Silver Casket Cool with Pearls,* by Edna St. Vincent Millay. She was a role model for me. I often wished that I could be more like her.

We met during our first year at Washington University. For one year immediately after college, she taught English and history in junior high school. We decided to marry at the end of that school year. When the Air Force called me to active duty, however, it meant postponing our wedding. So we decided to get married during my leave before starting flight training—only a few weeks away. June's teaching contract kept us separated for the next three months. During the next three years, our first two children, Frank and Kathy, were born, and we lived in Texas, Mississippi, Arizona, and Ohio. Away from parents and friends, we learned to rely on each other and became best friends.

Shortly after I joined IBM, our third child, Jeff, was born and we lived in Missouri, California, Ohio, Connecticut, and Virginia. After our children started college, June returned to school for para-legal training. Japanese friends spent a Christmas with us, and Saeko described June as the perfect role model for a woman who wanted to have both career and family. June managed our home and was the family nurse and sympathizer—the perfect caregiver. Alzheimer's disease began to creep into our lives sometime in her forties.

Chapter 1
Secrets of Survival

During June's journey into Alzheimer's disease, I experienced the trauma of losing my best friend, companion, lover, and wife—while still caring for her. The care requirements expanded as the years passed. So did the mental and physical strains. My experience did not equip me for my role. I slowly slid downhill emotionally. Armed with spirituality and determination, I began my struggle to survive the difficulties of around-the-clock care for a person with a long-term illness. An athlete all my life, I valued athletic metaphors: caregiving was not a sprint; it was a marathon. So I gauged my progress from year to year. After only partial successes at first, solutions began to emerge. They provide a map others may choose to follow, which will help them to deal more easily with years of sorrow and suffering. Some individuals may also need to seek counseling as a family member's disease continues.

The first few years, I was distraught and angry with June's behavior. Simultaneously, each year held new surprising developments. The middle five years were an emotional seesaw. Negative thoughts ruled my life until positive ideas temporarily overcame them. The down cycles started with each unexpected change in June's illness. At times, I found myself listing her irritating habits or those habits I resented. When baseball contracts were in the headlines, I wrote a facetious labor-contract for caregivers:

▸ On call—24 hours each day
▸ Regular pay—None
▸ Overtime pay—None
▸ Holidays—None
▸ Sick time—None at night, weekends or holidays
▸ Time off—None without a paid replacement
▸ Ambidexterity—Mandatory
▸ Needing more than two hands—Mandatory

I gained some relief by recording my negative feelings and the events that caused them. They resulted primarily from my lack of control over what was happening to June. Since I could not stop the progression of the illness, I thought about what I could affect.

The airlines say, "If you are traveling with a small child, please ensure that your mask is in place first. Then secure the mask for the child." To help June, I had to first learn how to "get my mask in place" for my emotional and physical challenges.

Using a lined sheet, I listed the following challenges (mostly emotional) across the top, and possible solutions down the side. Most of the solutions affected more than one challenge. After much testing, the solutions that remained became the *Rules* that helped me to survive.

ANGER

During the early phases, I had trouble controlling my emotions. Although I quickly recovered, I easily became angry. To overcome this tendency, I learned to:

Divert my energy

Keeping a daily journal allowed me to vent my emotions in a harmless way. My writings enabled me to analyze possible causes of my anger—usually a combination of fatigue and stress. Solutions to those two challenges also helped to eliminate anger.

Walking was not only healthy, but it also allowed time to think through a situation calmly. One may walk on an as needed basis, and as long and as far as strength allows. Gradually increase the frequency, the time, and the distance until it becomes an aerobic effort. By walking alone, one can also practice some form of meditation. While walking, one may also practice breathing slowly and deeply, and range-of-motion and posture exercises.

Keep a visible reminder

For each lapse of my control, I marked and circled an *X* on a calendar. Anger usually led to guilt, which yielded to remorse. These *X*s made me determined to manage my anger. As the solutions to my emotional challenges gradually took effect, the number of *X*s decreased significantly. It was uplifting to have a visual record of my progress.

Because my anger quickly subsided, these simple ideas worked for me. Someone who is chronically angry should seek professional counseling.

DEPRESSION

Depression came and went, but peaked when I had trouble coping with the realization that June had lost some of her capabilities forever. I lacked the initiative to follow routines, mostly reacted to the current emergency, and was unprepared too often. It helped to:

Maintain a positive attitude

Maintaining a positive attitude helped in fighting my way out of depression (and reducing frustration and stress). Inspirational messages helped:

▸ I Corinthians 13:13, "And now abideth faith, hope, charity, these three; but the greatest of these *is* charity."

▸ Sign on Episcopal Church: "God did not have time to be everywhere, so he created mothers." (I mentally added . . . *and caregivers.*)

William Faulkner: " . . . shall endure tomorrow and tomorrow and tomorrow."

Theodore Roosevelt: "the credit belongs to the man who is actually in the arena—whose vision is marred by the dust and sweat and blood; who strives valiantly, who errs and comes up again and again; who knows the great devotions, the great enthusiasms; who at best knows in the end the triumph of high achievement."

Henry Thoreau: "The mass of men lead lives of quiet desperation." (It encouraged me, knowing that Thoreau perceived that many others felt desperate too.)

Listen to inspirational music videos

Although few applied directly to caregiving, I grabbed any available support. These songs had memorable lines that seemed, as the Quakers say, "to speak to my condition."

From *I Will Stand by You*, sung by Corbin and Hanner

I'm not perfect, I'm no saint, Babe,

I don't wear angel's wings.

I'm no hero in shining armor,

All I am is what you see.

From *I Will Be There for You*, sung by Jessica Andrews, from the soundtrack of *Prince of Egypt*:

When I stumbled, you were right there.

For every act of love you've done, I owe you one.

There were hard times.

I know I survived just because you stayed by my side.

Change my focus

It helped to accept situations that had upset me in the past. The world never ended when I did not get things done on time or if I did not do them at all. (Health and safety were exceptions.) By being more accepting, I could then:

Focus on the positives. Instead of thinking about what June did wrong, I began to focus on what she did right. Saying positive things to her helped to reinforce my new feelings.

But have something good come from the negatives. Once a crown on a tooth came off less than a month after the dentist put it on. On the way to get it fixed, I stopped at Kinko's to get copying done. On the way home, I stopped at a Hecht's sale to purchase much-needed clothes for June and myself. As I gradually did more constructive things, I grew more confident and more at peace with myself. When I experienced more compassion for June and less pity for myself, I began winning the struggle.

FATIGUE

Fatigue affected me both physically and mentally. Four important rules helped:

Ambidexterity

When I did strenuous yard work, played sports, or moved June from place to place, it sometimes caused a physical problem. If I sprained my right arm, it resulted in nagging pains. Therefore, I gave equal employment opportunity to my left arm; I reversed hands for all caregiving tasks, and as many other things as practical. Any time caregivers feel awkward in doing a chore, that chore should be considered a candidate for switching hands.

After starting to feel comfortable using either hand, I began changing hands frequently. Sometimes I did half a task on one side with one hand and then changed sides to use my other hand (e.g., cutting her fingernails).

Pastimes

In his book, *Painting as a Pastime*, Winston Churchill said, "The cultivation of a hobby and new forms of interest is a policy of first importance. To be really happy and really safe, one ought to have at least two or three hobbies." So I gave up tiring and time-consuming pastimes. (This also greatly relieved frustrations.) That created the time for less-demanding pastimes, such as caring for wild birds. A computer game called FreeCell (solitaire) became a relaxing transition before and after caregiving.

Relaxation

My mental health also required other relaxation at least once and preferably twice a day. After getting June to day care and completing chores in the morning, I had a tea break and read. To cope with evening caregiving, I scheduled something relaxing just before June came home. After getting her into bed, I watched a movie. When I had even greater needs, I *wasted* the entire non-caregiving day, making sure that I did not do anything obligatory. (Some people could also benefit from meditation.) Feeling relaxed also helped to reduce anger.

Respite (the first of four survival cornerstones)

I desperately needed to get respite from continuous caregiving. In the middle of the companionship phase, June started going to day care, which enabled me to continue to care for her at home. My *recharged batteries* affected all of my emotions. The day-care facility provided a social atmosphere for June that was missing at home.

FRUSTRATION

In the early years, my frustration sometimes resulted in greater anger or stress. I needed to:

Accept risk

June sometimes got into mischief when I did not pay attention to her—an accident on the rug, eating soap or paper, hiding things. In the earlier years, I became upset when this happened.

Accepting infrequent situations that do not create a significant problem can reduce stress. If I felt that I could tolerate a bad result that day, I ignored minor happenings around me. As a result, I became much calmer and less stressed.

Accomplishing an objective made certain risks worthwhile. While I prepared dinner, I left June with food or a glass of juice in her hand, which saved me time. Spilled food or drinks became the cost of maintaining her ability to feed herself.

Lower expectations

June could not meet my initial high expectations. As I became more understanding, I set expectations at the lowest possible level, which she exceeded at times. As a result, I had more positive feelings about her actions. Instead of thinking about her lack of cooperation, I recognized her inability to cooperate. This also reduced my stress level.

GUILT

Guilt is a mantle most caregivers wear. To ease a feeling of imperfection, I needed to:

Provide care with dignity (the second of the four cornerstones)

Lumi Cavazos (Aunt Tita) starred in the movie *en Como Agua Para Chocolate* (Like Water for Chocolate). Others repeatedly asked her for the secret to her recipes. She answered, "The secret is that when you cook it, you do it with much love."

A year after I created rules for myself, I tried to put myself in June's place and wrote care rules from her perspective. From an original list of about thirty items, I focused on about ten.

▶ Allow me to use my abilities fully.
▶ Allow me to have areas where I may do as I please.
▶ Compliment me when I do something difficult.
▶ Continue familiar routines.
▶ Do not reduce my abilities with an overload of drugs.
▶ Do not discuss me in front of others as though I didn't exist.
▶ Let me move at my own speed.
▶ Smile at me and give me hugs.
▶ Treat me gently, with loving care.
▶ Treat me with respect and dignity.

These rules helped me become a more compassionate and effective caregiver and gave me peace of mind. They also seemed to raise June's contentment.

Simplify life

To find more time to offer care with dignity, I needed to simplify our lives. After a demanding life in the military and business, convincing myself not to try to be *all things to all people* was difficult. Gradually I came to accept this idea. My plan of graceful simplification included:

Companionship Phase

▶ Eliminating things June no longer enjoyed—for example, we stopped our joint social life.
▶ Giving away all houseplants.
▶ Preparing simpler meals.
▶ Stopping subscriptions to magazines and the weekday newspaper.
▶ Eliminating demanding hobbies, such as gardening.
▶ Reducing caregiving activities not related to health or safety (e.g., shaving under arms).
▶ Eating out together three times a week at local restaurants.

▶ Having a lawn service fertilize and spray the lawn and bushes.

▶ Having a cleaning service come once a month.

▶ Discarding or storing many things—June became more comfortable with less clutter.

Dependent Phase

▶ Reducing my tennis schedule.

▶ Approving many automatic electronic transactions for my checking account.

▶ Substituting biking for tennis because it could be done whenever I had free time.

Final Phase

▶ Stopping the Sunday newspaper.

▶ Simplifying holidays in stages by first not moving furniture to fit a tree and later eliminating a tree and celebrating at my daughter and mother-in-law's homes. I also eliminated decorations and lights on the mantle and outside, and I only put a wreath on the front door and a candle arrangement in the family room.

HOPELESSNESS

By the beginning of the dependent phase, I had a feeling of complete hopelessness. A few years later, subtle changes took place in me that I did not fully recognize at the time. I usually escaped by watching movies, but I could barely stand to watch any. Reading gave me less enjoyment, and I only did it while I had my tea. Even some of my favorite country singers lost their appeal. Although I had helped plan my grade school reunion, I decided that the long trip would be too much trouble. I missed the things I enjoyed most—companionship, eating out, and vacations. When I looked around the house, I felt pressured by the many things that needed doing. Finally, I became frustrated by my inability to lead a normal life. I desperately needed:

Something to look forward to

▶ It became important to have a form of hope. Our children helped by initiating a beach vacation in alternate years. Starting in the dependent phase, I could travel when June went to nursing facilities for two-week stays.

▶ After each event, however, I often had a letdown feeling. This led to planning a second event while I still enjoyed the euphoria of the first event. Having these events spaced several months apart kept me feeling hopeful.

IMPATIENCE

Pressures of an overwhelming schedule made me impatient, which resulted in feeling guilty. The demands of June's illness required that I learn to:

Manage time better

▸ To relieve the pressure of appointment deadlines, I planned to be early by a minimum of fifteen minutes.

▸ To save time, I saved short-duration jobs for as-available periods (during morning *quiet time* and between dinner and bedtime).

▸ I limited non-caregiving jobs to a few hours a day to allow for unexpected caregiving tasks.

▸ The day-care center closed on weekends, which demanded more of my time. So I scheduled my heaviest work for the early part of the week.

▸ I broke large tasks into preparation and execution, and then spread them over several days. Sometimes it took me six hours to mow the lawn; taking two days helped maintain my stamina for evening caregiving.

▸ In a slower period, I checked my calendar to see what I might do early.

INADEQUACY

At first, I felt helpless in the face of the staggering number of things I needed to learn. To avoid the demoralizing sense of being overwhelmed, I organized my efforts to:

Have a daily sense of accomplishment

Even in the worst of times, I could count on one accomplishment—I mailed a letter each day. This kept me in touch with friends, and ensured that I paid bills. It was also efficient because the mail carrier lowered the red flag when he came, which became my signal to check. On my better days, I produced more letters, so I saved some to mail on my worse days. Small accomplishments strengthened my resolve for larger ones.

After a time-consuming, difficult, or sweaty task (e.g., mowing), I often looked for a short, easy job (removing a few obnoxious weeds). Doing the unplanned five-minute job somehow gave me a greater sense of accomplishment.

From year five on, projects unrelated to caregiving kept me occupied mentally, physically and emotionally. First, I refinished two metal stair railings leading to the back yard, which held up for nine years. I averaged more than a half dozen projects a year. Most of them had a specific purpose: preparing our home for eventual sale, and making gifts for our children.

Starting in the dependent phase, I also began to feel proud of what I accomplished in caregiving:

- Restoring June's physical capabilities after her hip replacement
- Weaning her from drugs, which enabled me to renew her ability to use the toilet
- Maintaining her ability to feed herself
- Finding solutions to major challenges
- Caring for her at home throughout her illness

ISOLATION

At the beginning, a few persons seemed afraid of a disease they did not understand and rejected us. Accepting this rejection was easier than reaching out. With no one else in the house to talk to, I became a hermit. Sometimes, friends asked me to describe my life. I said I had the feeling of being down a deep, dark well; although I could see a small circle of blue sky, it seemed out of reach. I remedied the sense of isolation by:

Attending a support group (the third of the four cornerstones)

By the end of year six, I understood that I needed to share feelings and thoughts with others. In the middle of the companionship phase, I went to my first meeting of a support group. I recommend attendance from the diagnosed onset of the disease. Because of its frequency, the support group provided the companionship that I had lost.

Reaching out to family and friends

My tennis friends provided a great deal of moral support and a social life. When I had the time (and the need), I could initiate a function and they willingly agreed. As a result, we had lunch up to four times a year and sometimes took a RV on three-day weekends. When one of our group members built a large home atop Wintergreen Mountain, we began going there regularly. We usually stayed four nights. (It took me a day or more to *wind down*).

LESSONS LEARNED

- Do not wait for others to ask. Be the initiator.
- We could maintain a strong relationship in spite of the scarcity of our social contacts.

Notes

▸ Friends should make an offer to caregivers that they cannot refuse. It should sound something like this: "I have a couple of hours free next Tuesday morning. If you would like to get out of the house for a bit, I would be happy to come over."

STRESS

The lack of control over my situation caused most of my stress. In spite of the constant reminder of seeing things not done, I could not mentally juggle high priority items or get them done within a reasonable amount of time. As a result, I readily accepted handy solutions or what others told me, even when uneasiness told me I should not. One clue told me when I had lost control: I lacked time for a cup of tea. Managing time better helped to regain some control. I effectively relieved stress temporarily by:

▸ Doing mild stretching exercises.
▸ Lying down, closing my eyes, and relaxing my whole body for a few minutes.
▸ Immersing myself in music videos. In a stress *emergency*, watching *Desert Rhapsody* several times restored my mental health. (See Products Chapter.)

Three rules provided a more permanent solution:

Anticipation

Failing to anticipate could result in a messy room, a dropped drink, or a banana eaten with the skin. By the middle of the dependent phase, anticipation helped gain a semblance of control.

▸ It allowed me to redirect June into less-harmful activities.
▸ Looking ahead, I picked causes of stress that I could easily eliminate (e.g., I kept enough food and other supplies on hand so we would not run out).
▸ For times that had multiple causes of stress, I tried to eliminate at least one cause (e.g., I made early preparations for day care departures and arrivals, and for bedtime).

Flexibility

▸ When we had an early morning appointment, I shortened a less important function. For example, I cut her quiet time, but maintained her time in the bathroom.
▸ On bad days, I postponed scheduled activities so I could relax.
▸ If an unanticipated event delayed my starting dinner until it was time for June to arrive home, I ordered pizza.
▸ Sometimes, I had to postpone either a one-time or a repetitive

chore (mowing) of equal priority. I postponed the repetitive because it saved my doing it as often. That resulted in less stress and more free time.

▸ When near something that needed doing (and I could do it quickly), I usually did it. This was especially true if I needed to do it soon anyway (e.g., preparing fitted briefs for the next change).

▸ It helped to keep our options open. When June needed her hair done (though we didn't have an appointment), I still planned for it. Thus, I canceled day care transportation, arose early, and helped her get ready. Even if the stylist couldn't take her that day, I would only have to drive June to day care.

Solutions to major caregiving challenges

I started a haphazard list of New Year's Resolutions during the early years of June's illness. In a darker moment, I ranked a list of more than a dozen items entitled *Things I least enjoy*. Examples:

▸ Trying to get her to sit until she finished a meal.

▸ Four of the next seven items dealt with various aspects of bathing.

Writing these down motivated me to look for solutions. At the beginning of the dependent phase, I tackled the top items. I bought an adult highchair for her meals. The following year, I got a hand-held shower and a bath transfer bench, which greatly simplified bathing. By devising step-by-step solutions (a combination of products and improved caregiving skills), these lists virtually disappeared.

SPIRITUALITY

Spirituality affected all emotions. My parents grew up on farms. My siblings were seven and nine years older. During my five years alone at home during the day, my mother taught me her strong farm-practical religious values and philosophy. In resolving challenges, I naturally turned to:

Prayer (the fourth and last of the cornerstones)

In the movie, *How Green Was My Valley*, the minister (Walter Pidgeon) defined prayer as, "good direct thinking." Prayer helped me to admit my weaknesses, which led toward correcting them. During the early years, I prayed for wisdom, patience, empathy, strength, and the ability to give care with dignity. During the middle years, I added a prayer that I would not die first. (Not only did I feel that I could provide better care, but I also did not want others to have to assume the responsibilities.) In the final years, I prayed that June could die at home, without pain, and with me holding her hand. Even if God had not answered all of my prayers, they still gave me great peace of mind.

Visualization

My parents taught me that *God helps those who help themselves.* I often tried creatively to visualize how a different person might resolve some challenges. By removing myself from an emotional situation, I could think far more clearly.

THE TURNAROUND

Following these rules allowed me to achieve a better balance between what I did for June and myself. By the middle of the dependent phase, tangible signs of success began to show. In spite of the challenges that we faced, big changes took place in me. When winter storms cut me off from outside help for nine days, I easily rose to the occasion. This gave me great confidence in my caregiving abilities. Finding solutions to other challenges gave me newfound hope, and I saw more positive changes in myself. Instead of dreading three-day weekends, I looked forward to the extra time with her. When we took part in our last research study with the National Institutes of Health (NIH), I no longer needed to feel that it might provide a cure for June. Instead, I realized that we were providing hope for others. Contentment and laughter replaced negative emotions. Because of this humbling experience of being a caregiver, I became a kinder, gentler, and more spiritual person.

Chapter 2

Our Seventeen Years

Just as I did not notice our children's growth from day to day, I did not notice the gradual changes taking place in my wife. In retrospect, however, warning signs occurred. When she turned forty-one, we moved to the eastern part of the country. Although she liked to play the major role in choosing our homes, she left this choice to me. When she started a new para-legal job, she had uncharacteristic problems with the mathematics needed for real estate closings, and asked me to help. By age forty-nine, our children were away at college. When they came home, they recognized changes more rapidly. In talking to them years later, they wondered why their mother was becoming more forgetful.

Alzheimer's disease has no exact *schedule*, but many of its landmarks occurred in our journey of love, loss, and learning. By having some sense of what to expect during the steady deterioration, caregivers can prepare and plan, using our experience as a template. Instead of the medical definitions of Alzheimer's phases, *independent, companionship, dependent,* and *final* phases should have more meaning to a caregiver.

Independent Phase (Five years—did traumas accelerate the disease?)

June had an uplifting experience when she stopped smoking. Unfortunately, three emotional traumas pummeled her immediately afterwards—spaced only six weeks apart. First, her father died. Then she lost her para-legal job. Finally, an overwhelming trauma occurred for us; our younger son, Jeff, died in an automobile accident.

When June's former employer rehired her, she seemed happy, but he let her go again. During the first three years, she tried hard to continue with her life and find a job as a para-legal. She held two consecutive jobs in that field. The second firm kept her for nine weeks, but then they too released her. She gradually lowered her sights and trudged from one building to another, calling on any company that had an office. Her daily notes showed that she mailed résumés to hundreds of companies. After that, she held more than a dozen entry-level jobs, all for short periods. I learned to tell when a job was ending; she would say, "They were mean to me today."

Throughout this time, she retained her sense of aesthetics. Whenever she went out, she dressed and groomed herself well. She also had a quilt custom-made, for which she specified a beautiful combination of colors. Normal behavior deceived me into believing that little was wrong. Physical and emotional exhaustion put me into bed for four days. Comforting me brought out the best in June, and she seemed her old self. At the start of this phase, Christmas buoyed her spirits, and she did a good job of planning and buying gifts. She also bought a Weekly Minder that helped her keep appointments.

After it became obvious something was wrong, however, we started looking for answers. We turned to a neuro-psychiatrist. After four months of tests, the diagnosis: early onset Alzheimer's. We hadn't heard of the disease. Poised, June responded, "Thank you very much." As we learned more, we hoped to find some means of slowing its inevitable progression. After all, she was only fifty-three years old! We enrolled in drug testing programs at the National Institutes of Health (NIH). Although they had some onerous procedures, she willingly undertook them. We hoped that immediate improvements might come from the drug studies and that the research studies might yield a cure.

At the end of this phase, June still cooked simple meals once a day, did the laundry, cleaned occasionally, and visited with neighbors. She shopped for food moderately well, but it took several trips to buy all of the items we needed. She still rode a bicycle, but only with me.

WHAT TO EXPECT

June's first symptom was short-term memory loss. She had trouble carrying on two-way conversations, but cleverly covered up, either joking or changing the subject. Infrequent visitors said "I don't see anything wrong with her." After receiving answers to her questions, she asked them again a few minutes later. She constantly put important papers away for safekeeping and could not remember where. (I never found some of them.) Sometimes she brought in the mail and misplaced it. Only after receiving delinquent notices did I realize that something had gone wrong. Without running the dishwasher, she reused the dirty dishes and utensils. Repeated long distance calls to our son, Frank, included a wrong area code. (She forgot to use the homemade note pad and pencil board that our daughter put beside the telephone.) She bought, dated, signed, but forgot to give birthday, anniversary, and holiday cards. Forgetting that she already had a Weekly Minder, she bought a second one and made entries in both. Consequently, she began missing appointments. When she wrote checks, she could not always complete her name in cursive. She missed completing the check register and could not remember the payee or amount. Once after shopping, she could not remember where she parked her car. At the end of this phase, she made out an excellent Christmas list but forgot to purchase some gifts. In one Christmas card, she wrote "Love, the Fuerst family. We are pleased to see your success and happiness. Love, the Fuerst family." She wrote an appropriate thank-you note to our son and his wife, but she signed their name to it. She caught her mistake and rewrote the note, but forgot to mail it.

Her judgment also began to suffer. For a close friend's wedding, she bought a set of inexpensive drinking glasses. Returning from work, I sometimes found either (or both) the furnace or air-conditioner on with the doors and windows open. She continuously ordered vacuum cleaner bags. (Our huge supply outlasted the vacuum cleaner.) When charities called to ask for clothing donations, she gathered up an armful without regard for what she had. Most mornings, she arose early and brought in the newspaper. Now, however, she began delivering it to neighbors' driveways. Other times, she gathered up their newspapers and brought them home. When we applied for Social Security disability, the clerk asked June for permission to verify her statements with her doctors and former employers. She emphatically said "No," and I could barely contain a grin at the shocked look on his face.

Physical coordination became more challenging. She kept herself busy, but could not follow the routines in her jazzercise class. One minor car accident was not her fault, but she failed to take evasive action.

LESSONS LEARNED

Before diagnosis:

▸ Don't assume that changes in behavior are normal. Be alert to subtle clues (e.g., a family member saying, "I did something dumb today.") Document them to make it easier to tell a doctor.

▸ Choose a doctor for diagnosis who can distinguish between depression, menopause, and dementia. A neuro-psychiatrist may be more likely to recommend tests that will give a more accurate diagnosis.

After diagnosis:

▸ Get financial and legal affairs in order while your family member still has awareness.

▸ Enroll in drug trials, but keep expectations low.

Compensate for poor memory and judgment.

▸ Take charge of the checkbook. Give family members a weekly allowance. Fill out the checks, so they merely have to sign and cash them.

▸ Shop together, so she/he can still choose favorite foods.

Resolve safety concerns.

▸ To ensure assistance in case of driving problems, buy a membership in AAA.

Smell the roses.

▸ Write down good things about your family member. A prompt may be to list A-Z, and have a sentence for each letter. (Cheating is OK. X could stand for exceptional.) Start telling these feelings early and often.

▸ Cherish normal times. Birthdays, anniversaries, and other holidays may be the last your family member can fully enjoy. Try to make them special.

▸ Take pictures of each other, other family members, pets, and favorite places to add to a memory box for use throughout the years.

Companionship Phase (Three years—a time too short)

A few years earlier, we started talking about the possibility of my early retirement. June bought a book of house plans, and we both spent many hours looking at them. She did an excellent job of picking out the home she wanted. I retired in time for her fifty-fifth birthday.

Alone with me, June seemed content—especially if we did something that she liked, such as traveling or eating out. She also still had enough initiative to plant a flower garden. She introduced herself and greeted newcomers at the adult day-care center. Many thought she was a member of the staff. Because she had great empathy, she helped comfort those in need. She enjoyed holding Marissa (our first grandchild) affectionately. Sometimes, she talked about her condition. Almost ready to cry twice, she said, "I don't know why I act this way." These previously *normal* acts now seemed like accomplishments.

WHAT TO EXPECT

Physical challenges evolved into safety concerns. When I awoke early one morning, the garage door stood open as she returned home in her nightgown. Her scratches suggested she might have fallen into a thorny bush. A friend of hers, from a dozen houses away, later told me that she had knocked on their door. NIH staffers worried about her spatial relationship perception, which affected her driving ability. A neighbor confirmed their fears by telling me that she drove as if she were suicidal.

Anxiety appeared as a new symptom. June could seldom relax, and she paced the room like a caged animal. During the night, I could not sleep because of her restlessness. She seldom let me out of her sight and often clung to me desperately. When I locked myself in a room to study for an Italian language test, she pounded on the door until I let her in. Two couples that we knew well came over on New Year's Eve, but she felt uncomfortable around them. Although I made sure she always had at least twenty dollars, she repeatedly said, "I don't have any money." She developed an obsession about doors that closed automatically. Until they closed completely, she would not release them. The day-care center wrote: "Appears angry to be here and asks for her husband often. Her anxiety is unpredictable."

Her ability to do normal activities of daily living decreased significantly. First, things went wrong in the kitchen. She forgot how to make hamburgers and burned a roast to a crisp. June also had trouble buying clothes, so I went with her. When she came back from the changing room, however, she had trouble remembering which ones fit. She also had more difficulty deciding what to wear, so I helped her choose matching outfits. For a wedding, I chose a pair of panty hose. She became agitated at the reception and could not tell me why. After we came home and I removed the panty hose, I realized they were far too tight for her current weight.

Travel became more challenging. At crowded rest stops, June barged to the head of the line for the bathroom. At the end of one travel day, I laid down in our room for a few minutes. She walked into the room next door, then sat and talked to strangers as if they were old friends. Their shock did not allow them to react until she left. Staying with friends, she woke before me, went to their room and perched on the side of their bed, chatting away as they awakened. Multiple times, she arose in the middle of the night to go to the bathroom, became confused afterwards and crawled into bed with our hosts.

One of the saddest changes that took place was the effect that June had on our dog. He was part golden retriever, very friendly and always stayed near home. Our home had fourteen acres of forest in the back, so we let him run alone. Gradually, his behavior changed, and he barked almost constantly to go in or out. When a neighbor reported his being out without a leash, the police told me to stop. Walking our dog on a leash, however, gave her something enjoyable to do. After a neighbor rebuked her for letting our dog relieve himself on his lawn, she only walked him to the end of our short driveway and then back. Riley began to change drastically. He chewed his fur off and relieved himself on our rugs. When I took him to the veterinarian, he said that our dog had psychological problems that reflected June's behavior. A family friend, who managed a large farm, had just lost his dog. So our daughter took our dog there, where he could finally run contentedly. Occasionally, June missed him and said, "Where's Riley?" A picture of him became part of her special cache of photographs. Once, she and her mother went to a shopping mall that had a pet store. She spent the whole time holding a puppy. She became angry with her mother when she refused to buy the dog. Going home on the bus, she would not sit with her mother. She said, "I thought I would at least go home with a new puppy."

LESSONS LEARNED

Resolve additional safety concerns.
▸ Buy a medical ID bracelet.
▸ Selling a family member's car will be a gut-wrenching decision. A car represents independence, so empathy should be your guide.

Begin helping with activities of daily living.
▸ Take charge of the cooking, but make sure that it is a joint effort. Ask for advice and make her feel as if she is in charge. Gradually, do the more complicated jobs.
▸ Pick out clothes together from mail-order catalogs and try them on at home.

Put a pet's welfare first.

‣ Pets are wonderful for someone with Alzheimer's, but someone with Alzheimer's is not so wonderful for pets. Under our changed circumstances, finding a good home for our dog was kinder than keeping him.

‣ As an alternative, have pets visit or visit a pet. We made sure that June had many opportunities to get together with our daughter's golden retriever, Carmel.

Continue to smell the roses.

‣ If it is financially feasible, retire to spend full-time with your family member.

‣ Plan something pleasant to look forward to after an unpleasant event (such as a drug trial).

‣ Don't let lack of time cause postponement of trips to see old friends and relatives. En route, do not hesitate to ask someone to take your family member into the bathroom.

‣ Try to do all of the other delayed joint activities.

‣ Get out the photo albums and pick out favorites together. Keep these in a single album or box. Make copies in case some disappear. Look at the pictures together. Keep them on a nightstand as his/her special cache.

Start balancing caregiving with caring for yourself.

‣ To see doctors and friends safely, start using adult day care or hire a companion for your family member.

‣ If getting enough sleep is a challenge, consider sleeping in another room. This drastic change will naturally upset your family member, so empathy rules again.

‣ Go to support group meetings.

Dependent phase (Five years—major mental decline)

A member of the day-care center staff also worked for us as a home companion. She reported that June rarely spoke at the center. Sometimes, however, she made an uncharacteristic comment. Looking at the man next to her, she said, "I can't stand the way he smells." Once, she got on the bus to day care and said "Hello Jan" to the driver. As I left the bus, she looked at me and said with a tear in her eye, "Poor fellow."

At home, she spoke infrequently, but with awareness. One day, she asked my name. I said, "Frank," and asked her name. She said, "June! You knew that." When I sighed once, she asked, "Are you tired?" After I said yes, she said, "I am too." In response to my greet-ings in the morning, she might say, "Hi darling" with a big smile, or, "I love you." After accidentally kicking me once, she said, "Oh, did I hit you?" When she heard a woman described negatively on the TV, she quickly said, "No, she's not." Another time, I accidentally left her cover sheet off. She let me know with, "It's so cold." She complimented her mother with, "Oh, you're so pretty." After she dropped her grapefruit on the floor, she made me laugh when she said, "Not mine."

At the beginning of this phase, June used both fork and spoon and had a good appetite. She still fed herself about 90% of her food. When I missed getting the seeds out of oranges or grapefruits, she spit them out. Even near the end of this phase, she could still eat well and walk regularly. Her balance was excellent. Coming down the stairs, she required no physical effort on my part—only guidance and encouraging words. Music on TV gave much pleasure. After a song in a PBS Christmas special, she said, "That was good." One night, she hummed along to *Claire de Lune*.

WHAT TO EXPECT

Anxiety and behavior continued to challenge me. At the begin-ning of this phase, the day-care center staff said that she cried more and was becoming more verbally abusive, physically combative, and aggressive. Accompanied by a machine-gun kind of noise, she started screaming frequently. (Although she made the same noise at home, she did not scream.) One day, the staff reported that she yelled 95% of the time and they had to separate her from the group. Besides clutching other participants and staff, she showed anger by kicking. They also said that she continued to need constant supervision.

Activities of daily living continued to suffer. She became to-tally dependent on my help in using the toilet. Two years later, she became totally dependent on my help in bathing and dressing. Al-though she could still feed herself, she sometimes had trouble using the correct end of the fork and finding the food on her plate. She also might turn a bowl of food over, or throw it on the floor. She tried to eat anything reachable, including briefs, a map, soap, a Brillo pad, and the newspaper. (I had thankfully rid the house of plants a few years earlier.) Frequently, she got up from her chair and walked away after each bite.

Wandering became the newest challenge. It first happened at our favorite Italian restaurant. While I was distracted paying the bill, she disappeared. After frantically searching for her outside, I came back to discover her calmly sitting alone at a remote table, looking at a menu. Her second and final disappearance occurred at the grocery store. Although she stood at my elbow, I concentrated on picking apples. The police found her more than a mile away on the direct route to our home.

Two years later, the first challenges arose in her ability to move from place to place. When she walked unaided, she sometimes walked into a corner and did not seem to know how to get out. One day, she wrapped the cord of the blow dryer around herself and could not get free. When she sat in the rocking chair, the instability frightened her. Perhaps she was trying to maintain her stability when she clutched and did not release a towel rack until she had pulled it out of the wall. While I spent a vacation with our children and their families, June fell several times at a nursing home. At home, she wrapped her bed sheet around her ankles and fell. A worse incident shortly followed. In the middle of this phase, she entered a nursing home for a long stay. On one of my visits, the Administrator mentioned that June had tried to leave the home. When the staff tried to redirect her, she clawed at them. To counter her actions, they increased the drugs that she took. She then lost the ability to feed herself. Because of my concerns over her heavy sedation, I brought her home earlier than planned. A few days after returning home, she arose in the middle of the night and fell. She hit the wall with force and cracked a hole four inches in diameter level with her knee. I found her lying on the floor. She showed no signs of pain. However, her hip had fractured and separated and needed an immediate replacement.

LESSONS LEARNED

Relieve anxiety and control behavior.
▶ At the beginning of this phase, the day-care center staff gave signs that they might stop providing care because of June's behavior. So, our neuro-psychiatrist started her on prescription drugs. They proved effective in controlling anxiety, but her awareness decreased and she could not maintain continence.

Increase help with activities of daily living.
▶ Although bathing may be frustrating and unsuccessful for family members, shyness and habit may inhibit them from asking for help. By using tact and patience, however, one's help will eventually be welcomed. On the other hand, June readily appreciated my help with dressing.

Resolve additional safety concerns.

▸ The first identification bracelet that I ordered had an elastic band that made it easy to remove. Order one that has a catch that is impossible for someone with dementia to unclasp. Carry recent photos and give them to others providing care and to the police in case of wandering.

▸ Install keyed dead bolts on all doors leading to the outside.

▸ Childproof the bedroom of your family member.

Get outside help.

▸ Have a good team of doctors in place early. When our daughter and her family decided to sell their townhouse, I cleared our basement apartment for them to use while they built their new home.

▸ June's mother helped for six months. Later, a live-in nurse moved in. Both stayed with June while I played tennis up to three times a week.

▸ Expand the use of others caring for your family member to include Saturday adult day care and overnight respite stays.

▸ Sign up for transportation to and from the day-care center.

Buy helpful products.

▸ geriatric chair (the equivalent of an adult highchair) can re-strain someone during meal times. To my amazement, June liked it (possibly because the <u>day-care</u> center used them). It was the first product that I bought that solved a major challenge. That solution offered the hope that I could also solve more challenges.

Don't give up.

▸ Unless exercising, June was wheelchair-bound for four months following her hip replacement. I felt that it would be mentally uplifting for us both if we could eliminate it. Within the latitude that the doctor gave me, I extended her physical activities. I added a second trip up and down the stairs. Then we began short walks. In addition, I encouraged her to get in and out of the tub by herself. It was thrilling when I could finally send her to day care without the wheelchair! For the first time, June had a condition that I could do something about.

▸ June became mellower by the end of this phase, and her psychiatrist reduced her drugs. This resulted in an increase in awareness. Consequently, she could use the toilet for the first time in two and one-half years—a major accomplishment for both of us.

Final Phase (Four years—major physical decline)

After eight long years, June's agitation finally disappeared. As a result, her doctor allowed me to stop giving drugs. Uncontrolled movements disappeared, she began to use either foot to get into the bathtub, and she could initially traverse stairs. After she reached the top of the stairs, I usually said, "Good job." I varied this once with, "I am very proud of you." After waiting a few moments, June said, "Good job" to herself. Using the toilet regularly greatly increased her ability to maintain continence. The day-care center reported, "Enjoys exercising with the country music. Often reacts when looking at scenic pictures."

Through the third year of the final phase, June showed signs of awareness. She got herself into comfortable positions when sitting or lying down, including crossing her legs. Occasionally, she reached to hold my hand. The day-care center also reported that she responded well to music and conversation, and she smiled and laughed.

Even in her final year, she continued to speak irregularly but with awareness: "Yes" (after hearing Mary Chapin Carpenter sing *He Thinks He'll Keep Her*). "It's terrible" (while eating an unfamiliar soup). "Good" (while eating a familiar food). "Thank you" (when Bryan, our eight-year-old grandson, adjusted her geriatric chair and when I helped her into our car). "Don't" (when I accidentally knocked over something). "Sure" (when I asked if she wanted to watch television).

Also during that last year, our six-year-old grandson, Evan, said he had a scout project and asked if he could help her. I showed him how to get her attention and give her food and a drink.

WHAT TO EXPECT

Activities of daily living continued a downward trend. June moved more slowly and tried to step out or up as she came down the stairs. As I led her to the toilet, she sometimes confused it with the bathtub and tried to step into it. Shortly after that, she became totally dependent on my help in moving from place to place. She reluctantly pulled down her undershirt or blouse and seldom lifted her feet into shoes and slippers. However, she did continue to help raise her arms to undress. She spilled more drinks and became totally dependent on my help in eating. To illustrate the contradictions of this disease, one night June wiped her mouth very politely with her bib and then tried to eat it.

Following the elimination of drugs, she had an initial increase of awareness. Shortly after, however, a major physical decline started. Treatment of a foot ulcer took many months and was the most difficult of the medical conditions that I treated. The bus driver bringing her home from the day-care center had to use the bus-lift because she could not climb the steps. The grip of her left hand weakened. Day-care center staff reported that she was passive in most activities, needed assistance of a staff member for the range of motion exercised, and experienced a general decline. They reported tremors in her hands and feet. They thought she had a mild seizure and sent her home in a wheelchair. One week later, she had a fall that decreased her ability to traverse stairs. Then she had a mild seizure at home.

A vicious cycle began to occur. June's weakened condition required greater physical effort on my part. As I needed more rest, I increased the number of her nursing home visits. This resulted in a corresponding increase in urinary tract infections. That caused her to spend more periods in a wheelchair. After recovery, she was weaker than before the cycle started.

Her recovery from infections was complicated when she became resistant to both penicillin and sulfa drugs. When an infection made her too sick to go to the doctor, a visiting nurse team came to our home. They insisted that I put her in the hospital, but I felt that my personalized care would more likely succeed. Our doctor supported my view, and I justified her support.

Later that year, she had a violent seizure and blood issued from her mouth. Our doctor called the Hospice of Northern Virginia, and they admitted her that same day for evaluation and stabilization. After fifteen days, June arrived home in time for her birthday. Hospice staffers set up visits for five days a week and prepared me for the worst. I told them, however, that they would see a dramatic change at home. Although it took nine weeks, her eating, exercising, and ability to stay awake returned to normal. I could also give her a bath in the tub, she could use the toilet, and I could get her out of the house by myself. The pleasantly surprised hospice staffers discharged her from their program.

During her last four months, June could not help me in moving her from place to place. The exertion of getting her into the house caused me to lie down once. She went into a nursing facility for two nights shortly after that. During her final nursing home stay, she got another infection. Although she was barely conscious when I brought her home, I still felt optimistic. I told our children that drug side effects could be causing her lethargy, but I was wrong. I was happy that I could hold her hand and feel her spirit leave as she finally found peace.

LESSONS LEARNED

Continue to resolve safety issues.

‣ When traversing stairs began to take a long time, I worried about getting June out of the house in case of an emergency. So I moved her bedroom downstairs and set up the downstairs half-bath for her use.

Continue to install helpful products.

‣ Although we only needed to go upstairs once a day for June's daily bath, it eventually became too arduous. So I installed a stair lift.

Some descendants may not have known family members before they became ill. Try to leave these descendants with some positive views.

‣ It pleased grandchildren (aged four to nine) to do kind acts for their grandmother, and they then felt more comfortable with her.

Develop a philosophy on dying.

‣ Absorb the wisdom of one's doctors, nurses, other health care professionals, and members of one's support group.

‣ Anticipate future decisions. For example, if one wants a family member to die at home, make sure that is possible. If your family member would not want force-feeding, make the correct legal arrangements.

If one has some control over the inevitable, one can face it with greater serenity. The result can be an increase of one's own spirituality.

Chapter 3
Financial Concerns

Early onset dementia not only deprives a person of job-related income, but that person has neither retirement income from Social Security nor health benefits from Medicare. One should first get an expert diagnosis that will withstand scrutiny. Then apply for disability income under Social Security. The sooner one follows the ideas in this chapter, the greater the return.

Assets
▸ Have a record of all assets in a single place. A loose-leaf binder with tabs works well. Tabs may represent different types of assets and hold the latest statement. An introductory page for each tab may explain where more information may be found. List the contents of a safety deposit box and include a key to get into the box.
▸ It is time-consuming to retitle assets. Doing it as time allowed took seventeen months. If one plans to set up a trust, retitle assets afterwards to avoid doing it twice.

Early onset income
A person with early onset dementia may be too young to receive any retirement benefits. The working spouse may be in the same situation. This could place a family in a serious financial situation.

Determine your earliest possible retirement date. Then weigh spending the companionship years with your spouse versus the diminished income of an early retirement.

Calculate retirement income using several scenarios. To illustrate, assume these hypothetical monthly incomes: $1000 personal retirement at age fifty-five and $1200 Social Security retirement at age sixty-six.

Scenario #1

One could have a retirement income from age fifty-five to sixty-six of $1000. When Social Security is added at age sixty-six, the total would increase to $2200. The next two scenarios show how to increase short-term income, but at the expense of long-term income.

Scenario #2

Many early retirement plans have an option that allows a greater retirement amount until Social Security starts. Companies sometimes use the word *Leveling* to describe this option.

In this scenario, the greater personal retirement monthly income from age fifty-five until age sixty-six would be $2000. At age sixty-six, it would drop to $800, but Social Security would add $1200. Thus, the total would remain at $2000.

Scenario #3

One could also level a personal retirement plan to age sixty-six and take a reduced Social Security retirement monthly income at age sixty-two of $900. Personal retirement monthly income from age fifty-five until age sixty-six would still be $2000. At age sixty-two, Social Security would add $900 each month for a total of $2900 until age sixty-six. At that age, personal income would still drop to $800, and Social security would continue at $900 for a total of $1700.

Other considerations

Based on one's life expectancy, one should also figure the breakeven points of the various options. One can also use combinations of these scenarios. For example, one can level a personal retirement plan to age sixty-two and start Social Security at that age. Nothing is sacred about age sixty-two or sixty-six either. One can delay early benefits until after age sixty-two and delay full benefits until after age sixty-six. (Younger retirees will find that the government is increasing the age at which they will get full benefits.)

Get information from Social Security and your personal retirement plan. Substitute your information in a scenario of your choice. Many choices are available, so one may want to seek financial counseling.

Expense records

▸ Keep a manila envelope to hold expense receipts. Include any expense that one would not have had if a relative were not ill. Be complete; one can reject items that may not apply later.

▸ Keep an *expense* calendar to record items for which one has no receipts (e.g., medical mileage and tolls).

Income tax

Examples of ways to reduce taxes:

▸ Does the person with Alzheimer's qualify as a dependent? The IRS lists the tests to decide eligibility in the 1040 instruction booklet. IRS Publication 501, *Instructions for Dependents*, has details. Even someone who is not a relative may qualify as a dependent.

▸ Once a dependent reaches the middle stages of dementia, one will probably exceed the 7.5% of adjusted gross income required for a deduction of medical expenses. The 1040 instruction booklet section for Schedule A has an excellent list of the more common medical and dental deductions. A thorough list may be found in IRS Publication 502, *Medical and Dental Expenses*. Have a marker handy while reading these lists to highlight the applicable items. Then go through all checks and credit card statements for charges. Don't forget Medicare B deductions (from the annual Social Security statement, Form SSA-1099) and the year-to-date medical premium deductions from a year-end salary or pension statement.

▸ One may use Form 2441 (Dependent Care Expenses) to list the expenses of someone caring for a qualifying person so one may work or look for work. Depending on income, for tax year 2006, one could deduct 20-35% of the first $3000 of expenses.

▸ If adjusted gross income is less than $25,000, one should also investigate the "Credit for the Elderly or the Disabled." See Schedule R and its instructions for details.

▸ Under certain conditions, some states offer tax credits for caregivers.

▸ Because some laws change yearly, the IRS at 800-829-1040 can be helpful.

Insurance, Medicaid

Medicaid is a federal program administered by the states. A person must be sixty-five years old, blind, or disabled. Eligibility varies by state within broad federal guidelines, usually a combination of income and assets. A good starting point for information is the local Area Agency on Aging or an elder law attorney.

If one qualifies for a nursing facility, start looking early. Medicaid beds are often limited, and nearby facilities may be scarce. In addition, the admission's agreement for a facility may require the patient (or their agent) to pay full price for a minimum period. When a person enters a nursing home and Medicaid payments overlap with SSI payments, the latter are supposed to stop.

Insurance, Medicare

Medicare normally starts at age sixty-five. Disabled persons, however, automatically get Medicare Part A after they have gotten disability benefits for two years. Applying for Part B simultaneously is cost-effective. Health care providers automatically file claims.

The Medicare & You Handbook has a good one-page summary of Medicare Part A (Hospital), Part B (Medical), and information on all entitlements. Order additional booklets, such as Home Health Care, at 800-633-4227 (TTY at 877-486-2048) or go to www.medicare.gov and click on Publications.

‣ Part A does not cover long term care in a nursing facility, unless one requires skilled nursing immediately following a hospital stay of three days or more. Then, Medicare will cover the first twenty days and all except a daily deductible for the next twenty-five days. The daily deductible changes each year.

‣ Part B covers 80% of the approved amount for most health care and some durable medical equipment, but only covers 50% of the approved amount for visits to psychiatrists.

A doctor must authorize all durable medical equipment in one of two ways.

‣ Medicare requires a Certificate of Medical Necessity for a few items (e.g., hospital bed or wheelchair). Suppliers should then submit them to a Medicare Regional Carrier.

‣ Medicare will accept a physician's order (prescription) for other items (e.g., a geriatric chair). Suppliers have catalogs listing the items they carry. When one purchases a used item, however, one must file a claim with a Regional Carrier. A canceled check or a bill is adequate proof that one purchased an item. One must file a claim within one year of purchase, or Medicare will reject it.

LESSON LEARNED

‣ Be persistent in working through answering systems and regional staffs.

Insurance, private

Hospital

Hospitals automatically file claims. Some policies cover a skilled nursing facility for certain situations. For example, they may cover part of the daily deductible costs that Medicare does not cover.

Long-term Care

Since these policies are expensive and vary greatly in coverage, be a knowledgeable buyer. Determine the cost of each type of local care, including adult day care, home health, respite care, assisted living, and nursing homes. This will help to understand how much of one's costs one needs to cover with insurance. Then check the financial rating of potential companies. Use reference books (Standard & Poor's or A.M. Best) at the local library or check www2.standardandpoors.com or www.ambest.com. (Also read Chapter 9 and Appendix B in this book.)

Types of care
- ▶ What types does the policy cover? (Because hospice care is short-term care and Medicare covers its costs, it should probably have the lowest priority.)
- ▶ May one choose a subset of the types of care for a reduced rate? (If one plans on caring for a family member at home, a good subset would be day care, home health, and respite care.)

Restrictions
- ▶ Is skilled nursing care excluded?
- ▶ Are there penalties for pre-existing health conditions? (Do not consider hiding these. That will be cause for denying coverage or even policy cancellation.)
- ▶ What future health conditions, if any, does the policy exclude?

Qualifying for benefits
- ▶ Is prior hospitalization required?
- ▶ May a doctor certify one as unable to do at least two of six activities of daily living independently?
- ▶ Can one's own doctor provide that certification?
- ▶ What is the waiting (elimination) period before the policy benefits start?
- ▶ Is the waiting period based on calendar days or days of care? If it is days of care and one only receives care Monday-Friday, then benefits will start later.

‣ Is there a new waiting period for each level or type of care?

‣ If one has a temporary need for care, is there another waiting period for the next need for care?

Benefits

‣ Does one have a choice of getting payments based solely on one's disability, or solely on one's expenses, or for a set maximum dollar amount? If so, give this decision much thought. (Our situation would have needed eight and a half year's coverage.)

‣ Does the policy have inflation protection?

What about costs?

‣ Does the company guarantee that the cost will never increase? (The May 2004 AARP Bulletin cited a case of a 61% increase over a two-year period.)

‣ Is there an exception clause that grants the insurance company the right to apply to state insurance commissions for across-the-board increases based on total claims?

‣ What happens if one gets into a financial bind (such as the death of one spouse) and cannot afford to pay more premiums?

‣ If one starts to receive benefits, does one's payment to the company stop?

Other source for information

‣ One may also request a free long-term care consumer guide. Contact the National Association of Insurance Commissioners by e-mail at prodserv@naic.org or by calling 816-783-8300-2.

Major Medical

Companies may not provide coverage for psychiatrist visits beyond that covered by Medicare. On the other hand, they may pay for durable medical equipment not covered by Medicare.

‣ Even if Medicare says it will not cover an item, submit a claim to them anyway. Some insurance companies will not consider an item until Medicare has rejected it in writing.

LESSON LEARNED

‣ Be persistent in pursuing claims with an insurance company. (A hospitalization issue took more than seven months to resolve successfully.)

Long-distance caregiving

A close friend's parent lived on the opposite side of the country. In case of an emergency, not all children may be immediately available. Therefore, all children should have a power of attorney. The two siblings effectively handled this remote situation by:

▸ Setting up a trust through a bank in the parent's city. The trust officer visited the parent once a week to check on things and to provide spending money.

▸ Talking regularly with the trust officer.

▸ Automatically depositing Social Security and retirement benefits to the parent's checking account. The bank automatically deducted bills (including all utilities) each month. Because they had a joint checking account, the children could pay the few remaining bills.

Social Security

For all benefits, call 800-772-1213, TTY 800-325-0778, or go to www.socialsecurity.gov. One should get the literature for each benefit.

Disability Benefit

Even if one is too young to receive retirement benefits, one may be eligible for disability benefits. Family members should meet the conditions for being considered disabled if a doctor has diagnosed them as having dementia and they are unable to do any substantial work. In 2007, substantial work meant earnings of $900 or more a month.

It took four months to gather information and complete forms, and it took two months for Social Security to check the information and approve the application. (This did not cause a problem because payments do not begin until the sixth full month of disability.) Call Social Security to request:

▸ A Disability Starter Kit—one may also download this kit from the Internet.

▸ A Summary Statement of Earnings for your family member.

▸ The form entitled *Request to be Selected as Payee* (to request that the caregiver become a Representative payee).

▸ The form entitled *Statement of Claimant or Other Person*. This form allows your family member to designate a Representative payee. (The Social Security Administration did not recognize our Power of Attorney, but accepted this form as its equivalent.)

▶ A Disability Report. (One will need a complete employment record for the last fifteen years.)
▶ An appointment to file for disability benefits.

Retirement Benefits

If one-half of the well spouse's retirement income exceeds the ill spouse' disability income, the ill spouse should also file for retirement income.

▶ With an incurable disease, filing should be done early enough to start receiving benefits by age sixty-two.

Supplemental Security Income (SSI)

Those with little income and resources may apply for additional benefits. A house and car do not count as assets. If they get SSI, they may also be eligible for Medicaid, food stamps, and other social services.

Death Benefit

One must apply for the Social Security death benefit of $255 within two years. Only a spouse or dependent children are eligible.

LESSONS LEARNED

▶ Obtain a certified copy of your family member's birth certificate. The Department of Health in his or her birth state will send one.
▶ Find an original marriage certificate or obtain a copy certified by the custodian of the original.
▶ One will need copies of income tax returns and their supporting W-2s. Check each year on the Earnings Statement against income tax returns. For incorrect years, give copies of all W-2s to Social Security. (In our case, six years did not agree.)
▶ Wait until Social Security confirms that they have included the missing earnings with an Earnings Determination letter (or new Earnings Statement) before submitting a disability or retirement claim. (If they have not included all earnings, they will reduce payments.)
▶ Fill out the long Disability Report in pencil or via the Internet. (Making mistakes in ink is too easy.)
▶ Life will be simpler if one submits forms while family members can still sign their name. If they are unable to do this, take them along and file in person. That should prevent a rejected application.

Chapter 4
Legal Concerns

After diagnosis of dementia, getting one's legal affairs in order promptly is important. An excellent article on estate planning appeared in the December 2004 issue of the T. Rowe Price Investor magazine. Three pages explained everything clearly. One needs to take action while sick spouses are still fully cognizant and before they become inappropriately suspicious. Starting this process later is risky. These things have high priority:

▸ Have a family meeting with an attorney specializing in elder law. Having up to date information is vital because laws are changing rapidly in that area.

▸ If the ill person has the requisite capacity to conduct legal affairs, have them execute a durable power of attorney, including health care. Then update the wills of both spouses, in a way that will reduce taxes, no matter who dies first.

▸ Decide whether the assets warrant a revocable trust.

Advance Medical Directive

If a state allows advance medical directives, this directive replaces a living will and a health care durable power of attorney. In addition, the Hospital and Healthcare Association of my state published an excellent booklet called *Your Right to Decide* for its members, which included a simple fill-in form. The same form also allowed one to appoint an agent to decide organ donation. If a state does not allow advance directives, one may have to execute these documents separately. National Hospice and Palliative Care (800-658-8898) has an Advance Directive for each state. One may download a free copy at www.partnershipforcaring.org.

Living Wills

A living will concerns itself with a terminally ill person who may be in a permanent vegetative state or whose death is imminent. It should specify the limits of medical care. Most respite facilities asked for a copy. With fewer pages than the power of attorney, it made sense to execute and copy this document. Both spouses should have one.

A hospital or a physician in charge may overrule the provisions of a living will (*UC Berkeley Wellness Letter*, August 2004). So having a health care durable power of attorney is important.

Health Care Durable Power of Attorney (DPA)

This document empowers someone to decide health care for someone else, continuing in case of incapacity. The ill spouse should give this power to the well spouse. As insurance against the well spouse becoming incapacitated, both spouses should also give this power to a child or other relative. Our state allowed it, so we also recorded each DPA with them.

The American Bar Association (ABA) has published an excellent booklet entitled *Health Care Powers of Attorney*. One may purchase multiple copies of the booklet from them. Their address is 1800 M Street, NW, Washington, D.C. 20036. AARP also supplies single copies.

Choosing a lawyer

▶ Learn enough about elder law (including trusts) to speak to a lawyer. Sources: Day-care center classes, personal finance columns in the newspaper, the local library, and HALT (a nonprofit organization for legal reform) at www.halt.org.

▶ Pick a lawyer who specializes in elder law. Both the Alzheimer's Association and the Area Agency on the Aging provide information and referrals. The National Academy of Elder Law Attorneys (NAELA) at www.naela.org will provide names by zip code. Also, try AARP's Legal Services Network at 888-687-2277 or www.aarp.org/lsn.

▶ Speak to a potential lawyer by phone to learn his or her level of knowledge. For questions to ask, try the NAELA Web site.

Instructions to heirs

▶ After one finishes all financial/legal plans, have a page summary in case of death or incapacitation of the well spouse.

Include:
- Locations of financial and legal documents.
- Important phone numbers.
- Nursing facility preferences for both spouses.

Safe deposit box/ home safe
Important documents should be safe, but also accessible. To ensure availability when a bank or lawyer's office is closed (a long holiday weekend), one should store some documents in a safe place at home. Include originals of the advance directive (living will and power of attorney) and copies of wills or trusts. One should also give copies to adult children.

Trust, revocable
An excellent article entitled *The Multipurpose Trust* appeared in the August-September 1991 issue of AARP's monthly (then called Modern Maturity) magazine. Rather than willing assets to an ill spouse, it may make more sense to put assets needed for his/her care into a revocable trust. The person who created the trust pays taxes at their tax rate on any income from the trust. If the well spouse dies first, the ill spouse can receive income (and principal if necessary) from the trust. At the death of the ill spouse, a trustee can divide the remaining principal among heirs. A trust also eliminates the time and cost of probate.

Wills
One should rewrite all wills when creating a revocable trust. The will should have a pour-over clause to ensure that the trust receives any untitled assets. It took about two months to prepare a trust and two wills.

LESSONS LEARNED
- It could save time and legal difficulties if both spouses execute new wills shortly after diagnosis. Otherwise, the sick spouse's cognizance level may preclude executing one. Thus, one may only avoid inheritance taxes if the well spouse dies first.
- Before one transfers assets from joint ownership to single ownership, one should decide whether a trust is applicable. That will save transferring assets twice.

Chapter 5
Dental

By the fourth year of the independent phase, June started having trouble keeping her teeth clean. When her behavior became challenging at the beginning of the dependent phase, her periodontist of fourteen years asked me not to bring her back. Although we used Valium for calming, her regular dentist of fifteen years dropped her a year later. Using ideas described in this chapter, a new dentist provided care for an additional four years. Then he too felt that he could no longer cope with her behavior.

After that, even routine dental care required complete sedation. Only two dentists within a reasonable drive could administer it. After bad experiences with both of them, we made a long drive to a dentist who used an anesthesiologist. It cost more than $2300 to clean and correct several minor problems. June's doctor put a stop to dental care when she said that sedation was no longer safe.

Not enough dentists/hygienists have the skill and the desire to cope with many persons with dementia. As a result, the cycle of challenges and new dentists was frustrating and stressful. Using the techniques and products described here, one can provide reasonable care at home.

Teeth care

Independent Phase

Prevention is the best cure. Eliminate sugar from the diet. Brush after every meal using fluoride toothpaste. As brushing skills decrease, increase the number of hygienist visits to 3-4 times a year.

Companionship Phase

Encourage your family member by handing her the toothbrush with paste on it and asking her to brush. If that is unsuccessful, put it into her mouth and leave it dangling. That usually cues her to brush.

It also helps to put an arm around her shoulders while coaching. If she takes the brush out prematurely, say, "Here, let me help." (June usually thanked me and opened her mouth for me to finish.)

Dependent Phase

If uncontrolled movement is a challenge, a person will move less if seated. When she is tired and will not open her mouth, use verbal cues and slowly bring the toothbrush in at her eye level. To avoid having the paste wind up on a lip, insert the brush only when her mouth is open wide. To keep her used to the movements, wrap your hand around hers and move the brush together. This also allows her to feel that she is contributing and keeps her hand from interfering with the process.

Starting at the back is easier. Short strokes will ensure not bumping the back of the mouth. From either side, brush continuously until either top or bottom is finished. To reduce swallowing toothpaste, use pea-sized amounts of paste. Save the inside top teeth for last and brush that area as quickly as possible.

Final Phase

June did not completely clear her mouth of food when she swallowed. I tried both a Water-Pik and a toothpick with limited success.

Instead, pick a well-lit place where water is nearby. (With June in her geriatric chair next to the kitchen sink was easiest for me.) Wearing non-latex rubber gloves will reduce the danger that bites will cause flesh wounds. Slip a finger between the cheek and outer teeth to pull out food lodged against the outside gums and behind the back molars. This may take several tries. After being bitten once, I learned to insert my finger at the back corner of her mouth. Pull out large pieces (such as citrus skins) stuck between the teeth. Then use an Interdental brush (without paste) from the outside to clean between teeth at the gum line. To avoid hitting soft tissue, insert it only about 1/8 inch. (The brush will require frequent rinsing.) Give water before adding paste to the Interdental brush. The paste will stay on longer starting from the back (where the larger crevices are) and working forward. End with an electric toothbrush. With practice, one can reduce brushing time to six minutes.

Products to use

Electric toothbrush

If your family member stops helping to brush or becomes impatient with your brushing, get an electric toothbrush. A dentist recommended a Braun model. One may find various brands in groceries or pharmacies.

Advantages:
- ▸ This product was quiet and had a gentle soothing vibration. Its tiny brush head did no harm to areas where she had bitten herself. Even if teeth clamped down on the stem, the bristles still rotated and cleaned.
- ▸ It could do more in less time.
- ▸ When purchasing the toothbrush, also buy the inexpensive multi-pack replacement brush heads. Some stores also stock more expensive single replacement brush heads.

Interdental toothbrush

This tiny brush has circular bristles, similar to a bottlebrush. Interdental Brush and Proxabrush make them. The brushes lasted an average of seven months. A local grocery store sold a pack with a long handle with two brushes, a travel pack of three short-handled brushes, and a package of eight brush refills.

Advantage: This brush can get into the tiny spaces between teeth. Its bristles pull food out and clean in every direction. When flossing becomes impossible, this brush is vital. The tapered Proxabrush made access easier.

Products to avoid

Health care facilities or staff use or recommend products that work well for persons without dementia. Ask such facilities not to use disposable toothbrushes called Brushettes or Toothettes. They have flimsy handles and a plastic sponge instead of a brush. Unless one only brushes the outside teeth, someone with dementia can bite off the sponge and choke.

Persons with dementia swallow everything put into their mouths. The Poison Control Center said to swallow these three products created greater potential for stomach irritation:
- ▸ Mouthwash
- ▸ Toothpaste with baking soda and peroxide
- ▸ Prescription toothpaste is seven times as powerful as normal brands.

Other suggestions

Care Ideas

▸ Having the same dentist as your family member is more effective and efficient.

▸ Ask the dentist to check the entire mouth for sores from self-bites.

▸ If clenching or grinding occurs, consider a soft plastic tooth-guard (only worn at night) while the patient can still cooperate.

How to prolong use of a current dentist/hygienist

▸ Convince them that you can significantly calm your family member—perhaps by simply holding hands. This also keeps the hands from interfering with the process.

▸ To allow easier cleaning, suggest use of a bite block (rubber insert), which keeps the mouth open. Volunteer to hold it in place.

▸ Discuss the merits of giving a calming drug before visits. A dentist prescribed Valium (Diazepam) at 10 mg. June took it one hour before visits, and it helped.

Finding a new dentist

Look for a dental staff that has other patients with dementia. The best source is a local support group because members have first-hand knowledge of the care given to their family members. Other dentists or oral surgeons can probably supply more names. Make sure practitioners have personal knowledge of anyone they recommend. Ask the local Alzheimer's Association for a recommendation, but also talk to the person who originated the recommendation.

If the only option is sedation

▸ One may prolong treatment by your regular dentist if an oral surgeon is nearby. Discuss with them the idea of the oral surgeon giving the sedation and the dentist doing the cleaning and dental work. Let them work out a schedule for a joint appointment.

▸ Think twice about giving a general anesthetic for routine work. An option is to redouble your efforts on prevention, skip the routine exam and cleaning, and visit a dentist only for compelling reasons.

▸ Discuss costs of sedation in advance to avoid surprises.

▸ Make sure the practitioner has called your doctor to learn about the patient's overall medical condition before anesthesia.

Chapter 6
Medical

HEALTH PROFESSIONALS

Choosing a doctor

In their June 2006 report to Congress on early onset dementia, the Alzheimer's Association said, "When a person under age 65 goes to a doctor with symptoms of dementia, the doctor may not even think of dementia as a possibility or may not know how to diagnose it. As a result, getting an accurate diagnosis can be a long, difficult, and frustrating process." This process took us two years and nine months. If one suspects early onset dementia, one should choose a doctor who can distinguish between depression, menopause, and dementia. A neuro-psychiatrist may be more likely to recommend tests that will give a more accurate diagnosis. The best choice for most people is a doctor whom other doctors highly recommend.

In March 2006, the Mayo Clinic published the results of a study on what makes for an ideal doctor. The traits they listed were: confident, empathetic, humane, personal, forthright, respectful, and thorough. Their web site is www.mayoclinic.com. WebMD at www.webmd.com also reprinted the results.

Diagnosis for an early onset of dementia

After we finally saw a neuro-psychiatrist, it took four and one-half months to complete all of the tests. During that time, my wife made twenty-two visits to three doctors: a neuro-psychiatrist (the gatekeeper), a neurologist and a clinical psychologist. The duration of visits ranged from one-half to six hours. We also went to hospitals and an x-ray facility for a CT Scan, an electroencephalogram (EEG), blood/toxin tests, and various x-rays. All physical tests were normal.

Psychological testing evaluated her abilities, including memory, language, reasoning, comprehension, and perception (see Mental

Status Tests in Appendix D). These tests were not normal. They showed that she had significant organic brain dysfunctions, impaired cognitive functions, confusion, memory problems, and the inconsistency of having a sense of well-being but not knowing the date.

After eliminating all other possibilities, the neuro-psychiatrist concluded that she had Alzheimer's disease.

Drug prescription and monitoring

By the end of the companionship phase, the need for a drug solution became more pressing because respite organizations would not tolerate June's behavior. Guided by our neuro-psychiatrist, it took about nine months of experimenting with different drugs at different doses to find the best combination of antipsychotic and antianxiety drugs. At the end of the dependent phase, he said June was at the upper limit of the disease and had been at home longer than anyone he knew. We stopped seeing him when my wife stopped taking drugs. A person with that specialty:

▶ Sees many patients with similar disorders and can make an earlier correct diagnosis.

▶ Has an extremely high knowledge of current and future drugs.

▶ Understands the best dosage for a single drug and the interrelationship of multiple drugs.

▶ Experiments with different dosages of drugs to get the proper combination.

▶ Is most likely to know and recommend when a person should stop taking drugs.

▶ Is most likely to know about local research and know how to get a patient involved in those programs.

▶ Gives an appointment of thirty minutes or more, allowing one to plan an unrushed visit.

LESSONS LEARNED

▶ Have a team of doctors (a primary care physician and a neuro-psychiatrist) in place by the beginning of the dependent phase. Choose a geriatric specialist as the primary care physician. The team will probably expand later to include an orthopedic surgeon and a podiatrist.

▶ For the first visit to a doctor, bring a written chronology of other doctor visits, diagnoses given, and drugs prescribed.

▶ Continue to keep a log with key information about when adverse changes occur—behavior, temperature, various abilities (eating, drinking, sitting, and using the toilet). Bring a summarized update, reports from other doctors, and a list of questions to all visits. For urgent concerns, fax a report.

▸ Good doctors will more likely know and refer one to top specialists, when needed.

▸ Having the same doctor for yourself and your family member is more efficient.

▸ Think of your relationship with your doctors and their staffs as a partnership.

▸ Identify an authoritative staff person to talk to when the doctor is not available.

▸ Volunteer to calm your family member during any procedures.

▸ Ask your doctor to recommend disability plates. Get a temporary rear-view mirror tag until the DMV sends permanent plates. Getting June from the parking lot to her various appointments took much time. Because she could not take evasive action, it was also dangerous.

Hospitalization

My wife had two hospital stays. The first time, she could still walk.

LESSONS LEARNED

▸ The first hospital had no safeguard to prevent wandering. Rooms had a wide screen used for privacy, and I suggested the hospital put one at the end of the hallway where June walked. This simple deterrent caused her to turn around when she walked up to it.

▸ When transferring from one facility to another, ask to hand-carry medical records (especially x-rays). This will avoid having the same procedure done twice.

▸ Introduce yourself to the director of nursing, the nursing supervisor, the hospital administrator, and the social worker. Find out whom to contact for what. In case of an emergency, one will then know who to contact and where their office is.

▸ If a doctor operates, ask Medical Records for a copy of the operative report. It will be easier, quicker, and less expensive than trying to get it later.

▸ Inform all doctors, including a dermatologist, about a hip replacement. An infection in an entirely different part of the body may seek out a foreign material (such as a prosthetic hip) and cause a serious problem.

Ophthalmologist

One will only need this specialist during the first two phases. After that, a person with dementia cannot give the necessary cooperation and will not need reading glasses.

LESSONS LEARNED
▸ To lessen the chance of injury from a broken lens, buy plastic lenses.
▸ If a family member frequently loses reading glasses, find out what strength of over-the-counter eyeglasses to buy.

Visiting Nurses Association

As an alternative to a hospital stay, your doctor may authorize nurses to come to your home. (Your doctor should have a list of providers from which one may choose.) Based on the evaluation by the admitting nurse, nurses or aides may visit every day until they have resolved the critical situation. Medicare covers their visits.

HOME CARE

Bedsores
▸ If it is not against doctors' orders, an ill person should spend at least 50% of the day out of bed. Alternate between sitting, standing, and walking as often as practical.
▸ When in bed, rotate positions every two hours.
▸ Use a cushion to protect a heel; use a pillow or leg separator between the legs.
▸ Use an egg-crate pad and an air mattress with a massaging pump. (See Products Chapter.)
▸ Keep skin clean and dry. To increase blood circulation, massage areas most likely to benefit. Gently apply a skin cream daily on areas that touch or rub against anything (e.g., the upper spine and the back of heels).

First Aid

Ask doctors and nurses what to do in various situations. The American Red Cross also has excellent courses on how to handle emergencies until professional medical help can take over. In July 2006, they taught a three-hour course on first aid in my local area at a nominal cost. Call your local Red Cross office for a complete list of courses and prices. Also ask if they have a first aid textbook and a comprehensive first aid kit.

To treat some minor medical conditions (splinter or wound), one may need an extra set of hands to counter unwanted movement. If one is sitting, then one may hold an arm or leg gently between one's knees.

Seizures

Even a minor seizure can be frightening the first time it happens. Parts of the body may stiffen or jerk; a person may fall, and may also bite his or her tongue. Brightly colored blood in the saliva may appear. Minor seizures usually stop within a short time. Before a major seizure, several minor ones may occur, perhaps months apart. To prevent injury, get the person off their feet and stay with them until the seizure is over. Then call your doctor.

Urinary tract infection (UTI)

Prevention

According to the University of California, Berkeley *Wellness Letter* "Plenty of fluids may help prevent urinary tract infections." Doctors and health articles recommend cranberry juice.

▸ Buy the juice product with the highest percentage (usually 27%) of cranberry juice.
▸ Give a daily mini-bath using a hand-held shower.
▸ Read the section of this book about maintaining continence.

Detection

Enough liquids should cause pale urine. On the other hand, cloudy or strong smelling urine or an unnatural leaning to one side may show an infection.

▸ Take a urine sample in for analysis. Then see the doctor for an evaluation or antibiotics.

RESEARCH

Research is changing rapidly regarding causes, accurate diagnoses, and treatment. For the latest information, contact the Alzheimer's Disease Education & Referral Center (ADEAR) at www.nia.nih.gov/alzheimers or call 800-438-4380. ADEAR tells about the twenty-nine federally funded research centers, the three affiliated medical research institutions, and clinical drug trials.

Fortunately, the National Institutes of Health (NIH) (www.nih.gov) were within a reasonable distance from our home. At diagnosis, our neuro-psychiatrist said that he could recommend us to them. We worked with three of the fourteen institutes: the National Institute on Aging (NIA), the National Institute of Neurological Disorders and Stroke (NINDS), and the National Institute of Mental Health (NIMH). Our visits started in the independent phase and ended in the final phase. We made more than two dozen outpatient trips to NIH, and June spent more than six weeks as an inpatient for either research or drug studies (see Appendix E). NIH also offered four caregiver-counseling visits of up to two hours each.

NIH research studies

NIA had a rigorous screening process that consisted of questionnaires and personal interviews. June did an excellent job of filling out the admittance forms and a dozen pages of information. On the forms, she admitted to depression and that she had noticed changes with her memory. During the first stay, the PET (Positron Emission Topography) scan and the Magnetic Resonance Imaging (MRI) terrified June and she became exhausted. That stay confirmed that she had Alzheimer's disease.

Near the end of the companionship phase, she could not sign the admission form. Although she did not always know answers to questions, she effectively improvised. If doctors asked the month and year, she checked the calendar on the wall to supply the correct answer. We both became exhausted, and the staff agreed to shorten her stay from two weeks to one, but they still completed the higher priority evaluations and tests.

NIH drug studies

NINDS (www.ninds.nih.gov) conducted most of the drug studies. Their doctors were highly enthusiastic about the potential of each drug. All studies involved neurotransmitters (chemicals in the brain) that allow nerve cells to communicate. No drug worked for June.

Drug tests require a person to stop their current drugs about two weeks before a drug trial, continuing through the duration of the trial. By the beginning of the dependent phase, June became too dependent on her drugs to stop for the required period, which ended our participation.

NIH autopsy

Although diagnoses of Alzheimer's disease have become increasingly accurate, certainty requires an autopsy that reveals the formation of plaques in the brain. NIH consent forms contain the following statement: "It is important that an autopsy be done on those persons that we wish to continue to follow." The funeral home handled all of the details with NIMH, who did the autopsy free of charge. It confirmed Alzheimer's disease.

LESSONS LEARNED

▶ Research studies took a toll on both of us. Four years of intensive research became an emotional roller coaster of hope and disappointment. June had physical inconvenience, mental anguish, and did not like to be separated from familiar surroundings and me. One should take a break of at least six months between studies.

▶ Balance one's time between studies primarily for others (research) with those that might provide immediate benefits (drugs). Enroll in the drug trials, but keep expectations low.

▶ Research drug trials may provide immediate benefits for a participant. If a drug is effective, the manufacturers will normally continue to supply it free after the trial until it receives FDA approval.

END-OF-LIFE-PHILOSOPHY

Treatment questions regarding someone with advanced dementia

To decide treatment, one must consider moral, ethical, and religious values. An entire family should discuss the following starter sets of questions.

An example for all situations

▶ Would withholding the pneumonia vaccine be a kinder alternative for a terminally ill person?

When a person exhibits signs of awareness and wakefulness

Shouldn't one:

▶ Give diagnostic tests, antibiotics, and blood transfusions?

▶ Give intravenous fluids, oxygen, medication, or other therapies necessary to provide comfort care?

▶ Use experimental drugs?

▶ Operate if it has a high chance of restoring function (e.g., a hip replacement)?

▶ Cure a temporary condition even if it requires forced feeding through a tube?

When a person has few if any signs of awareness and wakefulness

At this stage, one may want to reevaluate one's thoughts regarding:

▸ CPR (cardiopulmonary resuscitation) for cardiac or respiratory arrest. An attending physician may fill out a DNR (Do Not Resuscitate) form.

▸ Intravenous fluids or artificial nutrition. Once one can no longer ingest food, is it too invasive to endure without a hope of relief except through death?

▸ Major operations, dialysis, cancer therapy, or blood transfusions. Might doctors save someone from one cause of death only to die a certain death from the primary illness?

▸ Whether or not to give pain medication may result in emotional conflicts. If pain is obvious, then one will want to give it. Keep in mind, however, that pain medication may cause persons to lose the little awareness they have and may shorten their life.

Immediate cause of death

Although Alzheimer's disease is fatal, members of the health care community and other caregivers say that the immediate cause of death can be a combination of side effects, such as:

▸ Pneumonia—often brought on by inhaling food or fluids.

▸ Starvation or dehydration due to the inability to swallow.

▸ Undetected infections, often originating in the urinary tract or kidneys.

▸ Failure of a vital organ.

Chapter 7
Prescription Drugs

June's agitation started gradually at the beginning of the companionship phase. To make her behavior tolerable to others, she started taking prescription drugs. Using trial and error, it took us more than two years to find a good combination of antipsychotic and antianxiety drugs. Both agitation and drug consumption peaked in the middle of the dependent phase. Then both declined at the same rate as they started—a bell-shaped curve.

DRUG TYPES (generic names are in parentheses)

Antidepressants
We tried three different antidepressants, but only had marginal results with them.

Antipsychotic drugs (neuroleptics)
In the companionship phase, we tried five different antipsychotic drugs. These drugs required a periodic blood test to check for possible liver damage. They resulted in uncontrolled movements (shuffling feet and mouth twitching), muscle rigidity, and backward arching. They also caused her to hold her arm up at a right angle.

At the beginning of the dependent phase, Moban (Molindone) controlled agitation well. Starting at a low dose, we experimented before reaching the best level. As June's awareness slowly declined, we stabilized her ability to function by slowly backing off to a lower dose. Her limited speech became more appropriate for the situation, and she became more helpful in dressing, eating, and other activities. Also, her hands became softer and less stiff and claw like. Along with these improvements, she had fewer happy moments.

We tried three different drugs to counter the side effects of the antipsychotic drugs. After experiencing their side effects with only marginal gains, we stopped using them.

Antianxiety drugs (tranquilizers)

Near the end of the companionship phase, June tried five different antianxiety drugs. The benefits were marginal, or they had too many negative side effects.

Early in the dependent phase, she started taking Klonipin (Clonazepam). With Moban, this combination worked well. The combination of low dosages of these two drugs made her less agitated and less easily distracted. For example, she finished eating food in her hand before reaching for more. Occasionally when she became severely agitated, I gave her an extra one-half dose. At the end of the dependent phase, we cut her dose in half. Within four days, her speaking ability improved noticeably and she ate faster, but her uncontrollable laughter increased.

DRUG SIDE EFFECTS

Most of the drugs caused loss of awareness and constipation. Other side effects included loss of libido, tremors, stiffness, and loss of appetite. As her awareness and abilities declined, it became feasible to reduce or eliminate drugs. Although it took about three months to see the full effects of a reduction in the antipsychotic drugs, we felt that benefits outweighed drawbacks. Nearly all of the side effects disappeared. Constipation, stiffness (especially her hands), and tremors decreased dramatically. She also had greater physical sensitivity, became more aware, remembered names, and could talk better. It took her less time to walk, she could dry her own hands, feed herself better and faster, and she provided more assistance during dressing. She regained the ability to clear her mouth with her tongue, and readily opened her mouth for me to brush her teeth. By the beginning of the final phase, we eliminated drugs. As a result, her ability to sleep diminished slightly.

LESSONS LEARNED

It is virtually certain that over the years, one will forget the side effects of a variety of drugs. One should record these side effects while they are still fresh in mind. (A one or two-letter code for the various side effects may reduce writing.) Understanding side effects when doctors prescribe several drugs simultaneously is hard.

▸ Ask the doctor what to expect and do if certain effects appear.
▸ Start only one new drug at a time. One should wait until one knows all side effects before starting the next drug. When changing dosage amounts, only change one drug at a time.
▸ Avoid adding a new drug and changing the dosage on another simultaneously.

GIVING PILLS

Preparation

Forgetting to give a dose is far more likely than giving too many. Put the drug information in a conspicuous place as a reminder (a lower stair for the morning pill, a coffee table near the TV in the evening). Set an alarm for a night pill. Start each week with a seven-day supply in a used prescription bottle to make it easier to track the usage.

Becoming confused when giving multiple pills is easy. Dedicate a calendar for recording doses until they reach a steady state. This is especially helpful when one makes a change in type or amount. Lay out the pills for each time of day. Other ideas:

▶ Adjust the pill schedule so a person is at home for all doses.
▶ Respite locations require that pills be in their original container, so save a used prescription bottle to send a supply to them for each stay.
▶ One will find it difficult to find partial pills mixed in with the whole pills, so save another used prescription bottle to hold partial pills.
▶ Use a pillbox that has multiple compartments.

What to buy

Anticipate that swallowing pills will become harder. Ask your doctor to prescribe sizes and shapes that a person can easily swallow. As swallowing those becomes difficult, try chewable pills, if available. As they become difficult, try a liquid, if available.

Giving whole pills

▶ Start with a small drink first. This eliminates a dry mouth, which causes rejection of pills.
▶ Hand them one at a time. As awareness declines, press the pill against a thumb, and the forefinger will automatically close on it. Then ask her to put it into her mouth. If that becomes a challenge, ask her to open her mouth and place the pill on top of her tongue.
▶ Give just enough water to wash one pill down. (This prevents drinking a full glass and refusing to wash down succeeding pills.)
▶ Check to see that your family member swallows each pill. Her mouth will open more readily if one approaches with a toothbrush or a spoon.

Chewable pills
‣ Put a glass of water into her hand and give oral prompts, which should trigger chewing.

Liquid medicines
‣ Stand to one side to avoid her accidentally knocking the spoon out of your hand.
‣ After giving medicine, fill the spoon with water and give that (to get the residue of medicine out).
‣ Use a small spoon to crush aspirins in a large spoon and add it to juice.

PHARMACY

A doctor prescribed Cipro (available only in non-chewable pills). Unfortunately, June could no longer swallow whole pills. Some pharmacies will not convert capsule-only drugs into a liquid form. Change to one that will. Our doctor recommended a small local pharmacy, whose pharmacist obligingly converted Cipro to a liquid form.

COST CONTROL

Some drugs can cost thousands of dollars each year. Even if one has drug coverage, expect problems getting reimbursement from an insurer. Try these ideas.
‣ Ask if a generic drug will do.
‣ If a drug is new or expensive, call the insurance company in advance to find out whether they will cover it. If not, contact the Food and Drug Administration (FDA) at 888-463-6332 to ensure that they have approved the drug for the use prescribed. Then get the doctor to write a letter explaining why this drug is necessary.
‣ Be persistent in pursuing claims with an insurance company. (A drug issue took me more than four months to resolve successfully.)

LESSONS LEARNED

To control the effects of dementia, work with a doctor to evaluate the type and quantity of drugs. Each drug should show benefits that outweigh its side effects. Progression of the disease may have the same effect as the drugs one gives, so also develop a plan with the doctor to reduce and eventually eliminate drugs.

For recurring curable conditions (such as urinary tract infections), use the least powerful drug that cures the condition. This keeps the more powerful drugs in reserve as a person becomes resistant to multiple drugs. The least powerful drugs also have better-known side effects and are the least expensive.

Some doctors started at the highest allowable dose or started low and quickly increased dosages. Although they planned to decrease later, the high doses created too many problems. Insist on starting with the minimum dosage. Be patient with this approach. Sometimes it takes longer (up to four weeks) to see results.

To understand the many drugs given by doctors and dentists, keep accurate records. One may find an accounting worksheet (42 rows x 16 columns) helpful.

▸ One worksheet could have a chronological list. It could include drug name, doctor, pill size, daily dosages, changes in a dosage, and start/stop dates.

▸ Another worksheet could show the time span covered by each drug. List drugs down the side and time across the top. Using a colored marker, highlight the time span that one gave the drug. This makes it easier to understand how drugs overlap, why certain reactions occur, and makes the data easier to explain to doctors.

▸ Another worksheet could group the drugs by type and compare expected results with actual results.

OTHER SOURCES OF INFORMATION

The best source about individual drugs (including side effects) is available at www.nlm.nih.gov/medlineplus, which the National Library of Medicine sponsors. This site includes Moban (Molindone), which I could not find elsewhere. Other sources:

▸ *The Pill Book* (See Bibliography).

▸ Consumer Reports maintains www.medicalguide.org for an annual fee.

▸ The Medical Letter, a nonprofit, at www.medicalletter.org is mainly for doctor use for an annual fee.

▸ Organizations around the country conduct clinical drug trials. Local chapters of the Alzheimer's Association have drug fact sheets. Some trials also advertise on the radio and in the newspaper. Besides the Alzheimer's Association, also check these web sites for drug trials: The National Library of Medicine at www.ClinicalTrials.gov and the Food and Drug Administration at www.fda.gov.

Other related sites

▸ American Society of Consultant Pharmacists, 1321 Duke Street, Alexandria, VA 22314, 703-739-1300 or 800-355-2727 or info@ascp.com

▸ Senior Care Pharmacists at www.SeniorCarePharmacists.com

GOLDEN OPPORTUNITY

Drug manufacturers should make patient-friendly medicines for persons with dementia. In order of preference, drugs should be in liquid form, chewable, or easy to swallow. They should make pills round, not too large, with a coating that makes swallowing easier.

Chapter 8
Products that Work

Some highly touted products work well for the physically disabled, but do not help people with dementia. The following cost-effective products all worked for me. Some products (labeled A+) solved major physical and psychological challenges. Knowing that they existed and buying them sooner could have relieved much stress. A few (labeled T) solved unique or temporary challenges. A few products helped me to lead a more balanced life. The author does not endorse any particular product. Use them as a starting point to do a comparative analysis with other products.

One can probably get many of these products free or at reduced cost. Put them on your birthday or holiday wish list. If a hospital or nursing home has charged for an item or they plan to discard it, ask for it. Check with your doctor and pharmacy for free samples. Ask your day-care center or support group what they might have to lend. Insurance may cover some products. Excluding clothes and disposable items, these products cost about $3000.

Bathroom grab bars

A grab bar gives confidence and reduces unwanted movements of a family member. A caregiver can also use one to help maintain balance. Buying and installing this product for a caregiver makes an excellent gift!

Types

Straight bars vary from one to three feet in length. Most local hardware stores also sell two feet by up to two feet *L* shaped bars.

Locations
▶ One vital location is on the long wall inside the tub so a standing person may easily hold it with both hands. Place a two-foot straight bar at a forty-five-degree angle.
▶ A two-foot bar may also be placed conveniently to aid in stepping in/out of a tub/shower.

▸ If the person with dementia is in an early stage, bars can aid in getting up from sitting in the tub and getting up from the toilet.

Installation

One will require a power drill, screwdriver, hole punch, stud finder, and a masonry drill bit the same size as the screw.

Bathtub mat, nonslip

If the nonslip surface of one's tub became worn, one may add a bath mat.

Bathtub transfer bench (A+)

Eventually, it will become a physical strain to raise your family member from a sitting position in the tub (number three of the things that I enjoyed the least). A transfer bench solves that challenge. Two legs fit inside the tub with suction tips, and two legs fit outside the tub. It has seat pads, a backrest, and may have a support arm on one side. The heights of the seat and the backrest may be adjustable. A person sits on the bench portion that is outside the tub and scoots inside the tub. The person remains seated for their bath.

Advantages

▸ Getting an extremely weak family member in and out of the tub will be easy.
▸ A caregiver does not have to bend over so far to help with bathing.
▸ The danger of falling disappears.
▸ The support arm helps prevent slumping.
▸ One may also use the bench outside the tub for brushing teeth, changing clothes, and eating meals in the bedroom.

Disadvantage

The seat pads only had a weight capacity of three hundred pounds—not strong enough for an occasional *plop* onto the seat by a 135-pound person. Replacement pads cost too much.

Recommendations

▸ One should research this product on the Internet. Two suppliers are Sammons and Graham Field.
▸ One should buy a bench with a minimum weight capacity of four hundred pounds.
▸ Make sure that the bench has a back and a seat that can extend

outside the tub.
▸ If one buys a seat without a pad, add a waterproof boating cushion.

Bibs (a much appreciated gift from June's mother)

A large dishtowel (15" x 25") did not work well as a bib. It came off too easily. One may tailor a large bath towel to a person. Make a neck hole three and one-half inches in from the center of an end. Then create two flaps above the neck hole and attach Velcro fasteners.

Advantages
▸ It catches most food if one stuffs an end under the place mat.
▸ The Velcro made them easy to use, and difficult to pull off accidentally.

Blood pressure monitor

Because of doctors' concerns about a drug's side effects, we needed a blood pressure kit. It measured systolic, diastolic, and pulses/minute. Before starting on the drug, we established normal rates at various times of day. Then we compared daily readings against the normal rates. One should research this product on the Internet. One site is www.portablenebs.com/bpmonitors or 888-255-2509.

Advantage
Using and reading it was quick and easy.

Blow dryer (an item we previously owned)

Look for these features: Multiple heat/blower settings and a washable filter. Avoid handle settings. (One may unknowingly turn up the heat.)

Clothes

Sort through existing clothes and separate those that one must dry-clean or hand wash. (Goodwill Industries will be a happy recipient of those items.) Have enough clothes to last at least a week in each season. By the dependent phase, expect to replace almost an entire wardrobe.

Look for
▸ Catalog availability
▸ *No-iron* fabrics that please the skin (no wool)

- Colorfast fabrics—fewer washing loads
- Warmth appropriate for current weight
- A limited range of colors: Solids and cream-colored tops will be more compatible.
- Comfort (including socks), but not so roomy that a person might snag a part
- Pullovers rather than button-ups save time.
- Tops with oval or V-shaped neck holes slip on more easily than those with round necks.
- Ease of fastening (no belts or zippers)—try elastic waistbands and Velcro
- Floor-length garments (pants, robes) should be short enough not to catch underfoot.
- Machine-washable in any water temperature—nursing facilities usually use hot water.

Avoid

- Dresses and skirts that reveal too much when they hike up while seated (or if the family member kicks her legs high).
- Shoulder pads

Footwear

Balance becomes a challenge in the second phase. Shoes with lower heels have a short life cycle. To reduce chances of falling, only buy flat heels. To ease a person's almost constant motion in the dependent phase, buy comfortable casual footwear. Men's tennis shoes have more room at the toes. Mail order catalogs have a variety of slippers. Both shoes and slippers should have non-skid soles.

Gloves

Thermal glove liners will keep hands warm. Mittens are better for curved and stiff fingers. One may attach them to a jacket with baby diaper pins.

Jackets

Get Velcro fasteners. (If an ill person fidgets a lot, others who provide care sometimes became impatient and ruin zippers.)

Nightgowns

- To compensate for tossed covers in the winter, use long one-piece flannel gowns.
- Buy those with flared cuffs. Sleeves with small hand openings or elastic at the cuff can slip up arms at night and cut off

circulation, causing hands to swell. They are also more difficult to get on. Ripping out elastic from a sleeve is a tedious job.

▸ For summer, order sleeveless, mail-order nylon gowns.

Pants/Culottes/Shorts

For modesty, order bottoms with solid crotches. Long pants (in two weights), culottes (knee length), and shorts work well. Because of changing waistlines, order those with elastic waists. Catalogs have them in a half dozen compatible colors with complementary blouses.

Socks

Overnight respite facilities have a knack for losing socks. Identification will show up better on light colored socks.

Undershirts

Undershirts add warmth in the winter. The boy's department of a department store has sizes that will fit a medium-sized woman comfortably. Since most undershirts will shrink considerably, buy the extra large size. They are easier to get on and will overlap fitted briefs. Wearing undershirts has other benefits. During a change of briefs, your family member can pull down on them instead of interfering with the process. Tucking a bib into the top of them is also easy.

Cups, spill-proof (T)

Spill-proof cups only dispense liquid when someone sips.

Dead bolts

One will find these bolts indispensable by the end of the companionship phase. To reduce the keys required, buy packs that use the same key. Get ones that lock the door from both sides.

Emergency signalers

During an emergency, one can seldom reach a phone. A friend's mother had a waterproof pendant signaler—light enough to be worn around the neck or wrist. By pressing a button, one may initiate two-way voice communication with an operator. Communication takes place through a master control unit attached to your phone. When one is unable to talk, however, the service provider immediately contacts the proper authorities. Signalers help in a long-distance caregiving situation.

Several companies manufacture signalers, including Life Alert (800-247-0000), Life Watch (800-716-1433) and various local companies with the name of Lifeline. These companies have a wide range of one-time setup costs and monthly fees. Ask about discounts based your membership in various organizations. The Federal Trade Commission calls this product a Personal Emergency Response System. For a free brochure, call 877-382-4357 and select option five.

Geriatric chair (A+)

By the dependent phase, someone with dementia will not sit still long enough to eat (number two of the things that I enjoyed the least). A recliner-type chair is too heavy and is not portable. A geriatric chair is like a wheelchair but larger and more comfortable. It should have a tray that can swing down out of the way. I bought a used one from a local distributor. (Had I gotten a Certificate of Medical Necessity from our doctor, Medicare would have paid 80%.)

Advantages

▸ It relieved the urge to get up and kept my wife seated in total contentment until she finished eating a meal. (Before purchase, find a day-care center that uses them and observe the effect it has on your family member.)
▸ Tucking the bib between the tray and the place mat will keep the area cleaner.
▸ The tray is a handy place to set drinks or hand-held food and decreases the chance that these items will wind up on the floor.
▸ Since the chair is self-contained and on rollers, one may eat meals in any room.

Disadvantages

▸ It is heavier and more difficult to take up and down stairs than a wheelchair.
▸ With both elbows on the tray, blocking the feeding process is easier for an ill person.
▸ It has small and difficult to use wheel brakes.

Glow-in-the-dark light switches

When one needs to turn on a light in a hurry, one will appreciate these. If they have not equipped your home with them, local hardware stores sell them.

Heel boot (T)

During the healing process of a heel ulcer, skin breaks down from pressure easily. This product protects a heel, but still allows air to reach the wound. One only needs to use it when a family member is lying in bed. One supplier for this product is Sammons.

Hospital bed

I borrowed a pre-owned bed. If not, Medicare could have paid 80% of the cost.

Advantages

▸ Side rails provide safety and peace of mind.
▸ The bed has rollers and is twin-size, so providing care from either side is easy.
▸ To prevent fluid from accumulating in a leg, one may raise the foot of the bed.
▸ To direct liquids at night, one may raise the head of the bed.
▸ Raising the head of the bed also made it easy to give drinks in the middle of the night.

LESSONS LEARNED

▸ A thicker mattress will be more comfortable for your family member, but then one cannot raise both the head and the foot simultaneously. This will cause some sliding when one only raises the head.
▸ It is longer than a regular twin bed and will require new sheets.

Hospital bed egg-crate pad

For a hip replacement, the hospital used an egg-crate pad as a mattress cover. It is more comfortable for a person who spends more time in bed than normal. Hospitals throw this pad away after discharge, so one should ask to have it.

At two different nursing facilities, June developed a bad blood blister on a heel. When one of them added the pad, the problem did not recur.

Incontinence briefs

Types

▸ Open-sided briefs (with elastic straps) do an excellent job in the early stage of bladder incontinence. They allow some airflow, which allows rashes and scratches to heal faster. On the other hand, they absorb less liquid. A wearer can also take them off easily, and they will not stay up if one has small hips.

▸ Fitted briefs (with tape tabs) wrap around the hips and eliminate those disadvantages.

Sizes

Medium and large fitted briefs have the same absorbent areas. Each side of the large size is three inches longer, however, which makes it easier to put on when bedridden. The large size is also more expensive.

Suppliers/Costs

▸ Generic brands cost half as much, but test them before buying a large quantity. I could not fasten one brand at the waist, so it sat low on the hips. That caused it to fall off once it absorbed liquid. Another brand had straps that easily came undone.

▸ Medium fitted briefs cost about 80% more than open-sided briefs. Large fitted briefs cost about 25% more than the medium brief.

▸ We got the best prices when our day-care center pooled orders for a sixty-day supply.

Incontinence brief insert

This absorbent insert lines the crotch of a brief. The extra absorbent kind costs more, but it keeps a person dry and dramatically reduces the laundry.

Incontinence draw-sheet

The size (37" x 37") of this washable absorbent sheet made it more useful than under pads, and its tuck-in flaps kept it securely in place. It came with a plastic bottom sheet as well. Using brief inserts and the draw sheet reduced laundry to about one-quarter of the previous amount. The Sammons mail-order catalog lists it.

Incontinence gloves, disposable

Doctors use them for examinations. Nursing facilities charge for these disposable gloves and only use a few, so ask for the partial boxes. Suppliers also sell them through catalogs. Make sure a person is not allergic to latex. Adenna sells gloves made of alternative materials. One can also look under *latex allergies* on the Internet.

Incontinence underpads

These disposable underpads have a waterproof backing. The absorbent area of the large size (19" x 29") makes them useful for a sitting area. By folding them in half, one can also use them on a car seat.

Leg separator or Adduction pillow (T)

This is a sturdy foam pillow 22" long and six inches thick. It tapers from fourteen inches to four inches. It has Velcro straps to hold one's leg. The hospital used it after a hip replacement. The product label said "*Span+Aids #50642-840 with band.*" Hospitals throw it away after one use, so ask for it.

▸ If a person rubs their ankles raw, keep this pillow between his/her legs at night to give the ankles a chance to heal.

▸ If choking is a possibility during the night, wedge it between the person's back and the side rail of the hospital bed. It keeps a person from rolling onto her back.

Massager, electric (an item we previously owned)

On the low heat and gentle massage settings, a massager can help to induce relaxation.

Mattress, air (and pump)

During in-home care, Hospice ordered an air mattress with a pump that caused the mattress to give a light massage and prevented bedsores. Home Health Clinical Services and Equipment Company distributed it, and Graham-Field, Inc., Hauppauge, NY 11788 manufactured it. Medicare covered its cost.

Mattress pads

These absorbent, washable pads (22" x 33") have a waterproof backing. If not using a draw sheet, one may overlap two of them at mid-bed atop the fitted sheet. They will prevent an entire sheet from being soiled. If one uses a draw sheet, one may still use these pads under the bottom sheet as a precaution. A woman from our support group gave me some she had obtained from a hospital.

Pill organizers

These plastic containers may have four compartments for each of seven days. Drug stores and catalogs sell them. (Suppliers also have Braille and beeper models.)

Pillow cover

These zippered washable waterproof covers keep pillows looking new.

Plastic covering

A roll of garden plastic is ten by twenty-five feet. It is stronger than a plastic mattress cover. Cut it to size and cover a bed before putting on the cloth mattress cover. One can also use it to cover a hospital bed before bed baths. One can find it at a local hardware store.

Runner, plastic (A+)

This twenty-seven-inch-wide runner kept our carpets in good condition. It had small plastic spikes on the bottom to hold it in place. One can buy it at a local hardware store.

▸ Place one on the side of the bed closest to the bathroom, one between the bed and bathroom, and others in the dressing and eating areas.

▸ To prevent tripping over it, place it where furniture can hold it down.

Safety support vest (T)

Justifying the use of a physical restraint is difficult. Use one only for a temporary period. During convalescence after a hip replacement, the nursing facility used a restraint vest to prevent further injury. One may also use it to avoid unanticipated problems in going off a strong drug.

To simplify donning it, the facility marked the back. Straps on the bottom front wrapped around and tied to the opposite side of the wheelchair or bed. A strap went through a loop to keep it from slipping.

Another type slipped over one's head and looked similar to a deflated life preserver. Both of its straps had loops to slip through. Others can become confused about how to put it on, so mark the front.

Advantages of the life preserver type

▸ One can easily get it on and off.

▸ On wheelchairs, one side could be in front of the occupant and the other side behind the wheelchair. Thus, one can easily put it on over a coat. Loops slip over the wheelchair handles.

▸ On a hospital bed, one may tie the straps where they cannot slip up and harm the occupant. To remember the correct location on the bed to tie it, draw an arrow with a marking pen on each side of the bottom strut.

Shades

Subdued lighting promotes calmness during quiet times. Installing opaque shades for all bedroom windows may accomplish this.

Shower, hand-held (A+)

This long-hosed shower replaced the normal showerhead. One can buy it at a local hardware store. Installing it is easy.

Advantages
▸ Because the caregiver can direct the spray, thorough rinsing can take place. Using one before soaping cuts down on the use of a washcloth. It does not irritate sensitive areas and reduces urinary tract infections.
▸ One can give a shampoo faster by not having to refill a rinse container constantly.
▸ On the gentle setting, the manufacturer (Teledyne) claimed a 70% reduction of water.

Spoon, measuring

Household spoons vary in size; variations in a dosage may cause challenges. These three-inch plastic tubes hold up to two teaspoons of liquid. The thin and brittle spoon purchased at a drug-chain splintered. (A local pharmacy gave thick sturdy ones away free if asked.)

Advantages
▸ Precise measuring
▸ No spills while carrying or giving
▸ One may prepare a dose and store it in the refrigerator for a few minutes until needed.
▸ A protrusion on the bottom allows it to rest so that the lip (spoon) does not touch a surface.

Disadvantage
A residue remained in the tube afterwards. (To insure giving the full dose, fill the tube with water and give that too.)

Stair lift (A+)

By the final phase, traversing stairs to take a bath was unsafe.

Notes

We would have had to add a shower to June's bedroom level. The stair lift was a simpler, faster, and less expensive solution. Since this is an expensive product, check the Internet. One site is www.silvercross-stair-lifts.com. One's goal should be to find a nearby pre-owned late model at one-third less than new. Don't expect to recover more than 10% of the purchase price.

Advantages

- The lift reduced traversing stairs from ten minutes to twenty-eight seconds.
- It eliminated the physical strain on me.
- When not in use, the lift only protrudes fourteen inches from the wall. Seat, footrests, and armrests fold up.
- A person can easily get into the swivel seat at the top and easily get out at either top or bottom.
- A seat belt prevented accidentally exiting.

Disadvantages

- The seat was high and difficult to get into at the bottom. It required physical repositioning.
- The footrest was small and too far back to tuck a person's feet on it easily.
- One cannot leave the lift against the stop in the fully up or fully down positions. It needs to back off from the stop to relieve the strain on the motor.

Supplies, first aid

- Alcohol (isopropyl) is useful for cleaning the one-second-ear thermometer's lens filter and for doctor-recommended wound care.
- Anti-inflammatory (e.g., Ibuprofen or Naproxen)
- Band Aids (especially the larger ones)
- Bandages (conforming 3" x 3.6 yards)
- Cola (decaffeinated)—make it *flat* (without bubbles) to combat nausea.
- First Aid kit containing larger bandages, gauze, compresses, and assorted items
- First Aid manual
- Gauze pads, sterile 3" x 3"
- Gauze pads, sterile non-stick, one and a half x two inches—the Johnson & Johnson brand was the most effective for freshly debrided areas.
- Ice-pack

‣ Ipecac syrup—call a poison control center before using.

‣ Milk of Magnesia (a mild laxative)

‣ Pain/fever relievers (Acetaminophen or enteric aspirin)

‣ Poly-sporin or a doctor prescribed ointment to prevent infections. The manufacturer stamps the expiration date in small numbers on the end opposite the tip.

‣ Tape, cloth, ½ inch x 5 yards

Supplies, other

‣ Baby powder (When a nurse saw me using baby powder in an area affected by incontinence, she said the powder became a reservoir for germs.)

‣ Baby safety diaper pins—use for items one easily loses (e.g., cap, gloves)

‣ Mild baby shampoo did not burn one's eyes.

‣ Baby washcloth, 100% very soft cotton

‣ Baby wipes—buy the Zip-Pak sealable packs, which do not need a container. If the wipes come in a container, save the container and buy the less costly refills. Since the generic wipes sometimes tore, I used brand names, which barely cost more.

‣ Bread wrappers, to dispose of used briefs

‣ Ensure Plus provided nourishment when swallowing was difficult.

‣ Gatorade helps to replace electrolytes when a person is unable to eat—try *Alpine Snow*.

‣ Skin cream: Our doctor gave a list, and Eucerin worked well for us.

‣ Soup (chicken noodle/rice)

‣ Straws, flexible drinking

‣ Zinc oxide worked well for a rash.

Suppliers

The author does not endorse any particular supplier. Use them as a starting point to do a comparative analysis with other suppliers.

‣ Adenna (medical gloves) www.adenna.com 888-323-3662

‣ Blair (clothes) www.blair.com 800-458-2000

‣ Dr. Leonard's www.drleonards.com 800-785-0880

‣ Graham Field www.grahamfield.com 800-347-5678

‣ Haband (athletic shoes) www.haband.com 800-742-2263

‣ HDIS (incontinence) www.hdis.com 800-269-4663

‣ Invacare (wheelchairs) www.invacare.com 800-333-6900

‣ Sammons www.sammonsprestonrolyan.com 800-323-5547

Thermometers

Battery-operated digital

It measures axillary (under the arm) temperatures. One inserts it in the armit and closes the arm over it. After two minutes, it gives a *finished* beep. To establish normal armpit temperature, measure it both in the early morning and in the late afternoon over several days. The digital readings varied no more than two degrees from oral readings.

One-second-ear

Accuracy came within one-tenth of a degree of an oral reading. To compensate for an occasional failure to point it at the eardrum properly, take several readings. Since each ear varies slightly, testing the same ear gives consistency. One brand is Braun Thermoscan (800-327-7226).

Toilet safety frame

This device helps to keep a person erect. Try using this device yourself for several days to understand its use. A few people or organizations have unused frames, so try to borrow one. If purchased, apply to Medicare for 80% of the cost.

Advantages
▸ The support bars allow one to reach back for support in seating oneself.
▸ If one has to use multiple toilets, its portability is useful.

Disadvantage

If used too early in the disease, the arms make it easy for a person to get up in the middle of using the toilet.

Toilet seat cover

Excessive scooting around on the toilet may cause an abrasion of the part of the spine that touches the toilet lid. Once skin care has cured the abrasion, a soft toilet seat cover should prevent it from recurring.

Transfer (gait) belt

These six-foot long belts fit around a person's waist to act as a restraint. During a hip convalescence, the physical therapist used one for walking and climbing stairs. They easily fit around a person and a wheelchair to prevent falls. Suppliers sell them through catalogs.

Urine specimen collection bowl

This plastic bowl fits under the lid at the front of the toilet seat.

Advantage

When one suspects a urinary tract infection, one can get a specimen to the doctor's office the same day.

Disadvantage

The front-to-back length of the bowl should be less, and the pour groove should be in front.

Walkers (T)

Following hip surgery, the physical therapist used a walker as an aid in helping to walk down linoleum hallways. Using it on the variety of surfaces at home is more difficult. However, it helps a person stand during some activities of daily living. (A friend's mother used a much-improved version that had a seat for resting and a basket to keep the hands free.)

Wheelchairs (A+)

During June's hip convalescence at a nursing facility, she spent her days in a wheelchair. For her return home, I borrowed a sturdy model with footrests and wheels large enough to go down stairs. One must periodically oil it and put air in the tires. Apply to Medicare for 80% of its cost.

Comparison with a geriatric chair

▶ It had smaller footrests and was lower by two-and-one-half-inches. Thus, one's feet can more easily drag on the floor.

▶ For eating, a lap tray would have been useful. If one has a handy friend, ask that person to make one that will snap onto the arm bars.

Wheelchair ramps

A solid surface ramp is wide enough for both wheels. A more portable kind has two lightweight (usually aluminum) ramps. They can telescope to fit the size of the steps and retract for easy storage. Each of the two ramps may have bumper guards to prevent the wheels from slipping off. Lengths vary up to ten feet. Support varies up to 800 pounds. One can find many suppliers on the Internet by searching "wheelchair ramp".

▶ One will not want to push a person up a steep slope. So, make sure the length of the ramp is suitable for the height of the steps.

Window locks

One may want to use these as a precaution to prevent wandering. They fasten the top and bottom halves of a window together where they overlap. They also act as weatherproofing because they eliminate any space between the window halves. A recessed screw requires a special key. Only one screw per window is necessary. Installation requires a drill, a 5/8-inch wood bit, and a ¼ inch drill bit.

PRODUCTS FOR A MORE BALANCED LIFE

Some products may ease one's life and enable one to be a better caregiver.

Telephone answering machine

A caregiver often feels isolated and cut off from the rest of the world. Calls are more important than for most people. Not missing a call that comes in when away from home greatly adds to a feeling of being connected. This product would be an excellent gift for a caregiver!

Telephone, Caller ID (T)

This product is useful during the early phases of the illness. That is when the ill person may answer the phone, but misplaces the message. One can usually obtain the caller ID box free during a sales promotion.

Telephone, cordless

At times, caregivers may expect an important call (perhaps from the doctor), but cannot leave the person for whom they care. By keeping this phone handy, they will not miss a call. In case of power outages, however, this phone will not work. At least one phone should be the old fashioned plug-in type. This product would be an excellent gift for a caregiver!

Telephone, mobile

If something happened to one's car while driving one's family member, it would justify having a cell phone. Select a phone small enough to carry on your person at home. If an emergency at home renders one immobile, one can still call 911.

VCR/DVD Player

Favorite TV programs will sometimes conflict with caregiving. A VCR allows one to tape and play them back at leisure. Also, during cable television outages (once for two days), one will appreciate having videotapes to watch. A DVD allows one to subscribe to a rental service, such as Netflix, that has a very large variety of films, including foreign films.

Videotapes/DVD

A videotape called *Desert Rhapsody* was hypnotic at times. Appropriate music accompanied wild flowers waving gently, pollination of flowers, animals grazing, dunes slowly shifting, sparkling streams, swans gliding, breathtaking scenery, vivid sunsets, rolling tumbleweeds, cascading waterfalls, churning clouds, and the splatter of raindrops. Once, June said, "It's beautiful." It helped relieve my stress. A set of half-hour tapes also included *Cosmic Rhapsody* and *Ocean Rhapsody*. The manufacturer also made a one-hour videotape and DVD, *Nature's Symphony*. Late in 2006, www.amazon.com or www.amazon.co.uk either had new or used copies of these products. Appendix A also has a list of other videotapes.

OTHER PRODUCTS

These sounded good, but I didn't use them

▶ One may apply inexpensive bathtub non-slip strips to the floor of the tub. Janitorial supply stores carry them. (Most modern bathtubs already have them.)

▶ Cord (electrical) shorteners are inexpensive plastic holders about five inches long with slots at each end. To help prevent injuries, wind excess electrical cords around them and hook the cords in the slots.

▶ Hip protectors act much like bicycle helmets; they disperse the force of a fall over a wider area and avoid impact to the hip itself. One product of this type is SAFEHIP® at www.safehip.com or 877-728-3447.

▶ Lifts may help transfer someone to/from either bed, bathtub, or car. If a physician prescribes it, insurance may cover 80% of the cost.

▶ Wireless baby monitors may keep a caregiver aware of activity in other rooms.

I used these, but they had questionable value

▶ An automobile swivel cushion has a wooden seat that is too hard for a long trip. In addition, it raises one's head almost three inches closer to the roof—a potential safety hazard.

▸ Vinyl mattress-covers tear too easily and are too difficult to get on and off.

▸ A pill splitter (designed for round pills) seldom cuts rectangular pills evenly, produces too many crumbs, and is not dishwasher safe.

GOLDEN OPPORTUNITIES

Donating most of these products proved difficult. Most nonprofit companies showed no interest in any products. A few asked me to bring the hospital bed to them, but it was too big and heavy. The Salvation Army only wanted the geriatric chair, but came to my home to get it. With the myriad of debilitating diseases, an opportunity exists for nonprofit companies to create a loan-closet. They could receive and distribute the larger, more expensive products used for home care. At minimum, it requires a storage facility and a volunteer with a van or truck. After the need for a product is over, most caregivers would be delighted that it could serve someone else. The loan-closet could inform people through support groups. In Georgia, Friends of Disabled Adults and Children (FODAC) already recycles some products for residents of that state. Since 1986, they have distributed sixteen thousand wheelchairs. Organizations in other states can find out more at 770-491-9014 or www.fodac.org/fodac/help. FODAC is at 4900 Lewis Road, Stone Mt. GA 30083.

The videotape that helped relieve my high stress levels (*Desert Rhapsody*) has not made the transition to DVD. Only eleven used copies are for sale. Since it would do much to help the millions of caregivers, producing that type of DVD should be profitable for a manufacturer.

Chapter 9
When Others Provide Care

Webster's dictionary defines respite as *temporary intermission of labor*. Getting respite was a cornerstone of my survival. To keep June at home for the entire length of her illness required the phase-in of appropriate resources. Using all of them showed me their advantages and disadvantages. Using more than one provider for each type allowed quality comparison. When a need occurs, one can then act quickly with the confidence that one is making a good choice. One should give all providers of care written helpful hints that will make their job easier. (See Helpful hints in Appendix G.) Continually update these hints and highlight the changes. Convince providers to use them to tailor their care. Tell them your family member will cooperate more readily if they do things as she is accustomed to having them done.

Independent Phase

It might seem that an ill person would require no care during this phase. With early onset dementia, however, one spouse is probably still working. That leaves the ill spouse alone during the day. Until the working spouse can retire, having a relative or someone else living in the home could be good. One may allow a provider of care to stay free in a spare bedroom in exchange for some services. Even if working or going to school, a care provider can fill some voids whenever the working spouse is gone.

Companionship Phase

As needs increase, one will need a greater amount of aid at specific times. For times during the day, day care is the most reliable choice.

Dependent and Final Phases

During these last two phases, one will need a blend of several types of care.

AT HOME

Live-ins

The day after our daughter and her husband moved out of our basement apartment, a student nurse moved in for two years. She kept June company so I could get away from the house at times. Depending on the services provided and the accommodations that one has, one may or may not pay them. (Appendix H has a sample live-in agreement.)

Finding one

▸ Young adult relatives may gain from living with an older person.

▸ These young relatives may also know nurses or someone in nursing school.

▸ Visit a local nursing school and let them know of your needs. If the nursing school has a bulletin board, see if they will allow one to place a notice there. Use tear-off strips with a name and phone number.

▸ Broadcast the need to one's day-care center, support group, and house of worship.

▸ The Foreign Student Service Council gives housing referrals and will list one's situation.

LESSONS LEARNED

▸ Thoroughly check the background of candidates. Do not choose one with a dependent. Their welfare will take precedence over your family member in an emergency.

▸ Do not allow them to earn extra money by simultaneously caring for others.

Other home care

At the beginning of the dependent phase, I seldom needed more than several hours of help and used reliable college students who lived in the neighborhood. When I needed longer respite periods starting the next year, I used experienced caregivers from agencies. To wrap around services that hospice provided in the final phase, I contracted with a company that employed certified nursing aides (CNA), who came for four hours a day. In a nine-year period, twenty-one different women stayed with June 171 times. Nine of those times allowed me to take trips. All companions had either technical caregiving skills or compassionate empathy, and some had both. Some of them left notes telling me what did or did not happen and whether it required action. (This helped if the companion took June to day care and was absent when I arrived.) They reliably picked June up or dropped her off at day care. If my plans altered, some stayed later than originally planned. One even disassembled my electric can-opener and put it in the dishwasher.

Advantages
▸ June stayed in familiar surroundings and received individual attention.
▸ One has no last-minute stress of packing belongings and taking one's family member somewhere.
▸ Holding a single person accountable is easy.

Disadvantage
If one pays a person $1000 or more a year, one has legal responsibilities as an employer (e.g., filing Social Security and unemployment taxes). Contact the IRS for the current law. However, agencies that provide home care assume these responsibilities.

LESSONS LEARNED
▸ When using a companion for the first time, ask her to come an hour or more ahead of your leaving. Show how one's family member is accustomed to getting help with the activities of daily living. Stay long enough to feel confident in leaving.
▸ If using an agency, make sure that they will send the same person each time.
▸ Post the do-not-resuscitate (DNR) order, medical emergency numbers, and helpful hints in a conspicuous place. A home companion wrote, "Her routine [helpful hints] that you have on the fridge is very helpful."
▸ Give companions directions to operate and reset appliances (e.g., the garbage disposal).
▸ If a home has separate heating and air-conditioning thermostats, label them appropriately.
▸ Put pills into clearly marked containers for each time of day. Lay out enough pills to cover your arriving home late.
▸ Anticipate a utility outage by laying out flashlights (and blankets in the winter). Provide emergency numbers for utility companies.
▸ As an absent host, one must anticipate all needs for an extra person. For example, find out the favorite foods of the companion and have them on hand.

AWAY FROM HOME

The easiest way to learn what care away from home will be like is by using a day-care center.

Day-care centers

Finding one

▸ Call the Alzheimer's Association to see if any day-care center specializes in persons with dementia. (A social worker at NIH recommended one that we used for more than ten years.)

▸ Check with the local county Agency on Aging about county-sponsored facilities.

Getting a family member to attend

▸ We convinced my wife that she would be doing volunteer work at the center.

Services to look for

▸ Do they sponsor a support group? Do they sponsor training? This could include talks on medical, legal, caregiving, and handling stress.

▸ Do they have separate programs for those in the early and later phases of Alzheimer's? An early phase program could have a peer support group and health education (including both physical and mind exercises) and a social group that includes the caregiver. A later phase program could provide participatory activities including cooking, crafts, discussion of current events, and group projects.

▸ Is there an exercise program?

▸ Do they have social functions that include the whole family?

▸ What are their hours? May one choose half days?

▸ What is their snow policy?

▸ Are they flexible enough to allow one to change one's schedule with notice?

▸ Will they give quarterly reports that could include weight, blood pressure, ability to do daily activities of living, and participation in group activities?

▸ Do they get samples of new products to allow users to try them at no cost?

▸ Will they pool orders of incontinence products so members can get a lower price?

▸ Do they offer flu shots?

Advantage

During the early phases, activities not available at home and social interaction with others stimulated June. During the dependent phase, art therapy, exercise, and singing raised June's quality of life. At the beginning of the final phase, they still experimented with a *memory box* filled with photos and other memorabilia that I supplied.

LESSONS LEARNED

▸ Take advantage of all training that they offer.
▸ Ask them to keep one informed of any change in your family member that they might notice. Do the same for them.

Nursing facilities

At the beginning of our journey, I had great doubts about my caregiving abilities. I did not decide then to keep June at home for the length of her illness. My thoughts about placement in a nursing facility fluctuated widely. Even a marathon runner knows that he has only about twenty-six miles to run. However, I didn't know how far I had to go and if I had the inner strength to get there.

Initially, I thought incontinence would cause me to place June in a nursing facility. When that challenge arose at the beginning of the dependent phase, the moment seemed to pass, and I didn't give it a second thought. At the end of that same year, someone asked when I planned to place June in a nursing facility. I said, "When I wear out physically." Early in the following year, I changed my answer to "When June wears out physically." If I could not transport her by car or bus, I could not get her to a doctor or respite facilities. Later that same year, I decided it should occur if I ever stopped feeling empathy for June. So the worries continued.

After I helped June recover from her broken hip, I gained the confidence that I needed. Then I knew I had the inner strength to finish our journey at home together. I had two fears: major physical problems for either of us and a loss of respite care. If I could successfully handle those situations, I felt I could succeed. The following year, I creatively tried to make my plan work. Ironically, that meant increasing the use of nursing facilities for respite.

Making the plan work also required a way to handle emergencies. A nursing facility reminded me of a lifeboat or life preserver on an ocean liner. It disconcerted me to think about having to use them. So did the thought of not having them available. If I could not successfully react to a major setback to June or myself, I needed a backup. So I approached a nursing facility with my concern. The coordinator assured me that a skilled nursing bed (at a higher cost) was usually available on short notice with the possibility of a custodial bed later. Knowing continuing care would be available gave me peace of mind and allowed me to complete my run.

Nursing facility types

Various types of facilities provide overnight respite care, including hospitals, nursing homes, and homes for adults (smaller, less expensive, less regulated, and with proportionally fewer nurses). During the last eight years of June's illness, nine different facilities provided an average of five days care per month. Some facilities had specialized units.

Alzheimer's unit

Half the facilities had a unit specializing in Alzheimer's. The best physical facility that I found had a separate house with a walled yard for residents. The house had three semi-private bedrooms surrounding a common area and kitchen. One nurse was always on duty. Because of the way the home set up its shifts, the residents didn't see more than five nurses.

The main advantage of these units is that most are secure and have their own staff. A disadvantage is that the facilities designed these units primarily for people in the earlier phases of the disease. Since some units exist in name-only, get a list of what is different. (Only one-third had special activities geared to Alzheimer's residents.) Security should include locked doors that a resident cannot open.

Skilled Nursing units

These may comprise an entire wing or just some beds in a nursing home. They provide a higher level of care, usually following a hospital stay. Medicare must certify these units to receive Medicare coverage.

Nursing facility experiences

Best experience

My mother stayed in the Lutheran Convalescent Home in St. Louis. Student nurses from the nearby Lutheran college augmented the excellent staff—all very caring. A chapel (and a chaplain) on premises meant that my mother could attend services regularly.

Second best experience

I first used overnight respite at Jefferson Hospital, and I was apprehensive. Although we only used them for only two days, I still stayed near my phone. As a first time user, I appreciated their telling me what clothing and articles to bring. They had a simple, fast, and reassuring admittance. The small, cozy ward only had eight beds, staffed with a RN and an aide. They took care of June four times, including a stay that allowed me to attend a twelve-day family wedding-reunion. No significant problems arose during the stays, and June and the aide seemed to get along well. Unfortunately, the hospital ended their program.

Third best experience

After June's hip replacement, her doctor certified that she needed rehabilitation. Immediately following her hospital stay, she entered a skilled nursing facility. Two days after she entered, I met with the dietician and the occupational therapist. I requested that they help her to gain weight, and regain mobility. They cooperated by adding super-nutritious cereal or soup to meals. After only two weeks, she gained weight and looked good.

Initially, her swollen right knee was bent and her right heel was off the ground. She had occupational therapy for two weeks and physical therapy for forty-five days. It took two persons to help with the physical therapy. In less than two weeks, however, she walked three hundred feet in a day. Three weeks later, she started climbing stairs. She did better going up than coming down. The nearby home and I had excellent communications, possibly because I visited twice a day.

Even with the wonderful things they did, one sour note appeared. One evening, I discovered one of her legs tightly wedged behind the highest front bar of her wheelchair. It is virtually certain that it could not have occurred after they seated her. The wrong type of movement would probably have broken her leg. Two strong staff members extricated her.

Worst experience

In the middle of the third phase, my stress reached a breaking point. Members of my support group highly recommended one home, and June went there for a long stay. Gradually, warning signs appeared. June had blisters on her feet, chapped spots on her face, had lost weight, and craved water. I met with the head administrator, who gave me lots of assurances, but said June was too agitated. To counter

June's agitation, the home initiated a calming medicine, and June lost more weight. Her breath began to smell badly. She frequently became constipated, and I found her dressed once without shoes, socks, and undergarments.

I became depressed and asked for a meeting with the owner of the home. At the meeting, I discussed my concerns, especially the rapid weight loss and the high drug dosage. In addition, I said I favored bringing her home. Three days later, the head administrator said the local doctor cut the drug dosage by one-third. Our neuro-psychiatrist, however, recommended an even greater drug reduction. Then I learned that the night shift tied patients into chairs, so I brought June home. The home had dehydrated her, she had lost twenty pounds, and her abdomen was hard and distended.

I had difficulty in seeing management of the home during that time as they brought records up to date for a state inspection. When the inspector came, the rest rooms finally had paper towels. The staff stayed on duty the entire time that the inspector stayed, and none of them ate until he left.

Second worst experience

The last year of the final phase, I took June into a home so I could visit friends and attend a writer's conference. When I visited her, she ate little, but drank a large glass of iced tea. Her lethargy caused me to suspect a urinary tract infection, and I asked the nurse to have her tested. It took them five days to give her an antibiotic, by which time her intake decreased to 50%. Three days later, she could not swallow food or drink. I could not help wondering how—or if— the nurse gave her the antibiotic.

Third worst experience

A nearby skilled nursing facility approached our support group and gave out certificates for a free night. June stayed there for seven nights while I went on a beach vacation with our children. When I brought her home, she smelled terrible. She had bruises (four inches in diameter) on both buttocks. My answering machine had two messages saying that she had fallen. When I called for the male nurse in charge, a nurse told me that the facility no longer employed him. It took several days to find someone who could explain what happened. The nurse said she had fallen four times starting shortly after I dropped her off, continuing through the day before I picked her up. She hit her head, buttocks, and elbow. (Our doctor later drained five and one-half cc. of bloodstained fluid from her elbow.)

LESSONS LEARNED

‣ I could tolerate sins of omission more easily than sins of commission.

‣ Except in rare situations, both physical and chemical (drug) restraints are affronts to a person's dignity and quality of life. Only two of the nursing facilities had a restraint consent form as part of the admission's agreement. They euphemistically worded the form and gave me oral assurances that the staff would only use restraints in an extreme situation. Unfortunately, one facility used physical restraints regularly as a punishment and to compensate for a lack of staff, especially during the evening and night shifts.

‣ Do not rely on government oversight to control nursing facilities.

‣ Have a withdrawal plan at the onset to enable quick action.

Nursing facility, finding a good one

‣ Check with one's religious or fraternal organizations. A nursing facility that they might sponsor is probably the best that one will find.

‣ If not, one may get a list of possible sites from Elder Care Locator, sponsored by the Area Agency on Aging.

‣ Ask doctors if they can recommend a facility.

Criteria to consider

Call each facility to ask questions and get literature, including a sample admission agreement. Ask one of them to include a standard condensed version of the Nursing Home Reform Law (OBRA '87). Then check these things:

‣ Rehabilitation ability

‣ Their availability of beds (preferably in private or semi-private rooms)

‣ Medicare-certification

‣ Are there qualifying conditions, such as age? (Only after spending much time talking to one, did I learn that my wife was six years too young.)

‣ Are there special arrangements for residents with dementia?

‣ What stages of dementia do they accept? (An extremely good nursing facility decided that June's illness was too advanced for their Alzheimer's unit.)

‣ Do they allow temporary stays?

▸ Is the minimum stay equal to or less than your needs? (Minimums usually range between two and fourteen days.) Ask about first-time use discounts.

▸ Security—for example, how do they prevent wandering?

▸ Safety—do they have a sprinkler system in case of fire? Do rooms have smoke detectors? On July 15, 2004, ABC News reported that one-third of the nursing homes do not have sprinkler systems and thirty-one persons in two homes died because of fire.

▸ Will they allow your current doctor to attend to your family member?

▸ How far in advance will they take reservations?

▸ What is the cost?

▸ An answer that starts with "We try to" should raise a red flag.

▸ A physical-restraint consent form should raise another red flag.

Initial visits (I visited about two dozen homes.)

▸ Visit at a mealtime. Talk to some residents, if possible. Do not become too entranced with a beautiful physical appearance.

▸ Check cleanliness and patient care. Eliminate those with poorly groomed, unhappy, or lifeless residents.

▸ Determine how long it takes to get there. (One may want to visit more than once a day.)

▸ Narrow the list and make unannounced visits during the second shift (usually three to eleven PM).

Other sources

▸ Nursing Home Compare at www.medicare.gov has information on quality measures, inspection results, and staff information.

▸ The September 2006 issue of *Consumer Reports* includes an analysis of sixteen thousand U.S. nursing homes. Of the homes in the country, they chose 4% to consider, and 3% to avoid. The site, www.consumerreports.org/nursinghomes, has state-by-state findings. For example, the state of Virginia had fourteen homes that one should consider and eight homes that one should avoid.

▸ The December 2006 issue of Reader's Digest had an article titled *Deadly Neglect*. Their checklist of what to look for when choosing a nursing home is at www.rd.com/nursinghome.

Nursing facility, preparing to enter

Questions to ask

▸ What documents do they require? Most want an original do-not-resuscitate order (if any), copies of a living will, a durable power of attorney, and insurance cards. Others want to see a Social Security card.

▸ Can one bring medicine and disposable fitted briefs? (It is less expensive if one can.)

▸ What hospital do they use in case of emergencies? (Check to see if your doctor has privileges there.)

▸ If your doctor cannot attend to your family member, is there a resident physician? (If not, ask what doctors have privileges there.)

▸ Do they provide bed rails?

▸ If they do not have a laundry service, will someone on their staff do it for a fee?

▸ Is there a VCR? Will they play music videos if one provides them?

Two weeks before admission

▸ Complete the application—usually about three pages long. (Since these take time, make copies for future use.)

▸ Stop changes in type or dosage of drugs.

▸ If they allow patients to bring their own medicine, have enough on hand to exceed the planned stay.

One week before

▸ A doctor must complete a medical history, physical examination (including an X-ray or test for tuberculosis), and a drug order. Have your doctor see to minor medical problems.

▸ Buy needed clothing.

▸ Tell the day-care center about the intended absence.

▸ For longer stays, get a haircut for your family member.

By the day before

▸ Make sure that you cut fingernails and toenails. (I forgot once, and they broke off the entire nail on my wife's large toe.)

▸ Cancel the day-care transportation for the duration of the stay.

▸ Update the care instruction sheets.

▸ Pack the easiest clothes to get on and off. Complete an inventory of clothing (see Appendix I). It is a reminder of what to pack, but it also helps in retrieving belongings.

▸ Place an identifying mark on clothing and other articles. (To decrease lost clothes, send light colors so the identification stands out more clearly.)

▸ At change of season time, try clothes on beforehand to make sure they still fit.

Day of admittance

▸ Allow at least four hours. One needs to drive to the nursing facility, sign the admission agreement (5-40 pages), pay (all want payment in advance), and get one's family member settled in.

▸ For good communications, get the telephone number for the nurse's duty station and the name of the charge nurse on each shift.

After admittance

Phone to see what the pill-dispensing chart says. Several persons may copy medicine data before reaching this chart. Twice I found it in error.

LESSON LEARNED

If the facility is too far away for your doctor, do not accept an offer from the facility to provide a doctor. The doctor may not consult you on his decisions.

Nursing facility care

All of the facilities tested well against questioning and initial observations. To ensure that the home is right for your family member, however, begin with one or more short stays there.

Assessing care

▸ Visit unexpectedly during various parts of a day, even at *no visiting* times. A good nursing facility didn't mind if I showed up during a meal to feed June. Meal visits allow one to see the quality of the food, whether care providers wash hands of other patients before meals, and whether they feed those needing help. One can also see how long people remain in restraining devices before and after a meal.

▸ Blend in with the surroundings in the dining room or a day room. Dress similarly to the participants and sit if others are sitting. Stay long enough so everyone forgets your presence. (To pass the time, we sat near a television and held hands.)

▸ Listen to what the care providers say to and about the patients. (One told a patient to eat faster because she needed to feed someone else. Others spoke unkindly about the patients.)

▸ Ask lucid participants about the way that the facility treats your family member.

▸ If possible, compare the usage of incontinent products to your usage at home.

▸ See if nurses will respond to reasonable questions or requests. If one is uncomfortable with an answer, get a second opinion. (One nurse said a deep, rumbling cough was a symptom of the disease. A second nurse said it suggested drainage, and it was good that it was loose.)

▸ Introduce yourself to other regular caregivers. Ask if they would like an update on anything occurring to their family member. If they are receptive, ask them to do the same and exchange phone numbers.

Negative indicators
▸ Physical restraints
▸ Lots of leftover food for those unable to feed themselves
▸ Signs of hurried or sloppy dressing

Expressing concerns
▸ Ask questions about what is normal, what they can change, and how long it will take.

▸ Anticipate problems, discuss a plan to avoid them, and pinpoint a responsible individual.

▸ Do not assume that each person in the chain-of-command is speaking to the others. Get to know the director of admissions, case manager, director of nursing, station head nurse, and charge nurse. Nurses' aides provide most of the caregiving. Talking with them may result in more personalized care.

Nursing facility summary

One should try enough facilities so that one can make a comparison. I had these feelings of comfort with the ten facilities that my family used:

Very comfortable—	two
Comfortable—	two
Acceptable—	three
Uncomfortable—	one
Very uncomfortable—	two

Based on our experiences, most nursing facilities did these things:

Well

They bathed their patients regularly, dressed them appropriately, kept enough clean clothes on hand, administered medicine appropriately, and moved residents from place to place safely.

Not well

Most of the homes were short of staff. When emergencies consumed the staff, they abandoned normal care. Because of the variety of people providing care during three shifts, they recognized and reacted slowly to changes in a patient's condition.

- None did a good job of maintaining skills and assisting with enough exercise. When I brought June home after longer stays, she temporarily lost eating skills and strength.
- None worked at maintaining continence, such as allowing a patient time on the toilet.
- Seven of the nine homes caused an injury (blisters, cuts, sores, and falls), or an illness. A blister on a heel or a raw sore on the spine suggested that she had been left in bed too long. In addition, she frequently had severe chapping of the areas around her mouth, chin, and nose. This cleared up after about four days at home.
- Most of them did not give enough liquids or provide complete incontinence care. In combination with little exercise, this led to constipation and urinary tract infections. Although June spent only 18% of the time in nursing facilities, 85% of the infections occurred there.
- Although they served enough food, June suffered a weight loss at four. At three, the aides lacked the time or patience to help in feeding adequately. (The fourth facility did not allow visitors at meal times.)

Costs

Monthly costs change so rapidly that one should check with Elder Care Locator to get comparative costs. Although a semi-private room daily rate at a nursing facility is high, extras usually drive the total daily rate even higher.

- Temporary stays could cost more than $30 extra at one-fourth of the facilities.

‣ One-third had one-time charges for shampoo, lotion, wipes, and washbasin kits. (Take the unused items home at the end of the stay. Several washbasins, for example, will be useful in giving bed baths.)

‣ Almost half had a daily service charge for hand feeding and incontinence.

‣ More than half required that they give medicine from their pharmacy and charged up to three times more.

‣ The most onerous charge is what I call the *extra night* charge by one-third of the facilities. They charged for both the days of admittance and discharge, even if a person only stayed for the end of one day and the beginning of the next. One can, however, bring one's family member early the first day (usually after breakfast) and pick them up late on the second day (usually after dinner). Even so, they save the labor of the two most difficult times of day (morning bath and breakfast on the first day and bedtime of the last day). What might one say to a hotel if one checked in at noon and checked out at noon the next day and found they had charged for two days? If using this kind of nursing facility, a longer stay will spread the extra cost.

‣ Although many charges are irritating, look at the total cost and make decisions based on that.

‣ Once one establishes a pattern of overnight respite, negotiate for multiple respites each year at a reduced cost.

LESSONS LEARNED

‣ Much of the care is dependent on the lowest paid, least trained, and most transient people.

‣ Even in the best of nursing homes, if a less-caring person has responsibility for your family member, poor care can result.

Respite care summary

Advantages

‣ A caregiver has time for chores, relaxation, and social functions.

‣ Longer respites allow a caregiver's minor sprains to heal.

‣ The time with one's family member is of higher quality.

‣ It enables caregivers to keep family members at home, where providing care that maintains their dignity is easier.

Abilities of a good care provider or facility
▸ Anticipation of needs
▸ Recognition of a developing problem or emergency—few problems are spontaneous.
▸ Wisdom to realize that tailoring care for each person simplifies their job.

LESSONS LEARNED
▸ Adult day care is the most effective form of long-term care. To make it work, however, one needs to intersperse both short and long overnight respites.
▸ If one plans a stay-at-home vacation, choose a nursing facility rather than home care. It will be far more relaxing.
▸ Fewer but longer periods of overnight respite are more helpful.
▸ A longer trip will be far more relaxing if one takes a family member the day before leaving and picks her up the day after returning.
▸ One cannot count on any single source of overnight respite. The best people or nursing facilities are in high demand. They also prefer a steady customer versus a sporadic one and longer periods versus shorter periods. Keep multiple backups for each type of service.
▸ Facilities rarely commit very far in advance for temporary stays. When one has a personal plan with a firm date, waiting until the last week for confirmation is stressful.
▸ When away from home, participants pass illnesses around, similar to schoolchildren.

Respite cost summary (Appendix J has a yearly percentage breakdown of costs.)

Decide what percentage of after tax income is affordable to spend on respite. (In my case, I averaged 25-30%, peaking only once at 35%.) Since 1997, one may deduct respite as a medical expense, so one may get part of that money back.
▸ For the same number of hours, using a day-care center is more cost-effective than home care.
▸ Using a combination of a day-care center and a nursing facility is more cost-effective than only using a nursing facility.
▸ Using an outstanding day-care center ten hours a day, five days each week may cost as much as most nursing facilities. However, some centers turn away no one for a lack of funds. (They cover fees through Title XX funds of the Older Americans' Act and scholarships. They fund meals under the Older Americans'

Act, and their cost is recovered based on ones' income.) In addition, those who do not qualify for scholarships can reduce the hours per day and days per week to an affordable level.

▶ The cost of longer overnight nursing facility respite is the same as a combination of weekday day care and weekend home companions (through an agency).

▶ Individuals charge 15-35% less than agencies for home care.

▶ If one has a rental basement apartment, analyze whether it is more cost-effective to rent it and purchase home care when needed. (In my case, I could buy 67% more home care with the rental income.)

OTHER SUPPORT

Day care transportation

Our county's Area Agency on Aging provided transportation to adult day-care centers for a reasonable cost. One must wait from one to two weeks for enrollment.

Advantages

▶ It allows one to have an extra hour of free time each day.

▶ Getting a wheelchair-bound person on a bus is easier than into a car.

LESSON LEARNED

June presumably arrived home from the day-care center at 4:30 PM. For various reasons, the bus sometimes brought her home more than an hour late, when both the day-care center and bus transportation office were closed. If they had not brought June home by 5:00 PM, I called the day-care center. I found out what time she had left and how many people had boarded the bus. I also obtained the after-hours telephone number of the bus dispatchers.

Hospice care

Hospice care emphasizes providing pain relief and comfort during a terminal illness. Most care takes place at home. The number of days will vary, but starts with an initial period of ninety days. After that, hospice administrators may approve an additional ninety days. Then they may approve more thirty-day periods. The hospice has an excellent handbook that clearly defines their services and what to expect from them. The handbook has sections on pain management and care ideas. A one-page contact list lists hospice 24/7 phone numbers, management names, and spaces to write names of the primary nurse, social worker, home health aide, and volunteer.

Acute care unit experience

Following a seizure, an admitting nurse recommended the acute care unit for evaluation and stabilization, and June stayed there for fifteen nights. The physical setting was beautiful, full of light, peaceful, and had an excellent cafeteria that visitors could use. The unit made life pleasant, and I learned about some products that we used for the remaining nine months that June lived. Their full-time staff of doctors and nurses was skilled, and caring. A social worker helped me find daily home care to wrap around the care that hospice provided. Shortly before death, care may take place in an acute care unit or in a nursing home or hospital that provides hospice care.

Home care experience

After the acute care unit, care continued at home for seventy-three days. The assigned nurse was extremely competent and caring. She came once a week, coordinated all other care, and reviewed monthly the written care instructions for the home health aides. Once a day, a home health aide came to give June a bath. A physical therapist evaluated June at the beginning and instructed me at time of discharge. A social worker provided the name of a volunteer and helped coordinate some end-of-life activities.

Costs

For Medicare to pay for hospice, a doctor must certify that a person is terminally ill. The person elects hospice care instead of standard Medicare benefits, and a Medicare-participating hospice program provides the care. Medicare helps pay for drugs for symptom control and pain relief (co-payment of $5 for outpatient prescriptions) and medical and support services. They also pay for up to five days of inpatient respite care every ninety days (co-payment of 5% of the Medicare-approved amount), and grief counseling after death.

For more information

Contact the National Hospice and Palliative Care Organization help-line at 800-658-8898. Their Web site is www.nhpco.org. It contains much information, including six frequently asked questions.

Long-distance caregiving

As my mother reached her eighties, my sister set up Meals-on-Wheels for her. Volunteers delivered a hot meal Monday-Friday for a reasonable fee. (It is also comforting to know that someone visits regularly.) When she needed more help, two granddaughters moved in with her. Although both worked, they gave help with day-to-day personal activities, shopping, and cooking. The next year, my mother needed someone around constantly and moved in with my sister. When that became too difficult the following year, I found a nursing home for my mother in St. Louis, our hometown. Using Eldercare Locator, I established criteria and defined a geographic area. Eldercare contacted the local Area Agency for Aging who sent me a list of three nursing facilities and the name of the local long-term care ombudsman. Getting information in advance will shorten one's time away from home. I chose a facility that lived up to all of my expectations, and it was only five minutes from my brother's home. Since I went to St. Louis frequently on business, I could see my mother regularly.

A close friend's eighty-six year old mother lived on the opposite side of the country. This is how the two siblings effectively handled this remote situation.

Early phase

▸ The mother wore a device, with which she could signal an emergency team for help. (See Emergency signalers in Products Chapter.)

▸ The mother enjoyed getting letters and kept the enclosed pictures prominently displayed.

▸ The siblings talked regularly with the mother and each other.

▸ They employed someone to clean the house regularly.

▸ The siblings, a spouse and two grandchildren all visited regularly.

Middle phases

▸ Initially, a care provider stopped by for less than an hour four or five days a week. She primarily provided food and social stimuli. Gradually, this became a team of two providers. Their visits increased to about four hours every day and included care in other areas.

▸ Siblings and care providers talked regularly.

Final phase

Since the mother wished to stay in her own home, she needed around-the-clock care. A lead from a church resulted in a team of two live-in care providers (one for weekdays and one for weekends).

For the final month of the mother's life, the doctor arranged enrollment in a hospice program.

LESSONS LEARNED

▶ Call the local county Area Agency on Aging to find out about local services.
▶ To encourage a parent to call them, children should consider having an 800-number.
▶ Make sure the care providers know what they should do in an emergency.

Other ideas

▶ Assisted-living-facilities have no standards for their services or staffing, so the U.S. Senate Special Committee on Aging commissioned a report, presented in April 2003. To learn more check www.aging.senate.gov.
▶ For a fee, a care manager evaluates a situation, makes recommendations, may arrange for services, and keeps one informed. Although this is more expensive, it may be the only option for some families. Eldercare Locator or the local Area Agency on Aging can probably give referrals.

Chapter 10
Other Resources

A caregiver can better survive caring for a family member by accepting help and actively seeking resources before needing them. Each resource will be part of a chain leading to others. Set a goal to use half these resources within a year after diagnosis.

Alzheimer's Association

The Alzheimer's Association invests heavily in research on the possible causes and cure of the disease. They also have many brochures. An excellent program that they sponsor is *Safe Return.* (See that topic in this chapter and Wandering in the Other Tips Chapter.) More than two hundred local chapters sponsor local programs and publish newsletters. For example, the National Capital Area chapter sponsors a day-care center that has a full-time director and a well-trained staff. (June attended for more than ten years.) They especially designed the day care for those with Alzheimer's. The chapter help-line also provided names of attorneys.

For more information
▸ Call their Helpline at 800-272-3900. Their mailing address is 225 North Michigan Avenue, 17th Floor, Chicago, IL 60601.
▸ Their Web site, www.alz.org, provides drug fact sheets.
▸ The local Alzheimer's Association may also list their number in the business pages of the telephone book. (The chapters near me are the National Capitol Area at 703-359-4440 and the WV Chapter at www.wvalz.org or 304-343-2717.)

Alzheimer's Disease Education & Referral Center

This center is associated with the National Institute on Aging and provides free publications on aging and Alzheimer's disease. Contact them at P.O. Box 8250, Silver Springs, MD 20907-8250, www.nia.nih.gov/alzheimers or 800-438-4380.

American Association of Retired Persons (AARP)

AARP has many publications, including a magazine that contains pertinent articles. Contact them at www.aarp.org or 1909 K Street NW, Washington, D.C. 20049.

American Health Assistance Foundation

Call 800-437-2423 or write 15825 Shady Grove Road, Suite 140, Rockville, MD 20850. Their programs include:

▸ Alzheimer's Disease Research—their web site, www.ahaf.org, includes brain illustrations, memory games, current research, scientist comments, and a chance to ask written questions.

▸ Alzheimer's Family Relief—offers limited financial assistance for respite, day care, medicine, or personal care of a loved one. To qualify, a caregiver must show financial need and provide a physician's statement of the diagnosis. Once qualified, a caregiver may re-apply every ninety days.

▸ They have many excellent booklets.

Area Agency on Aging

During the early stages, this county agency helped find other support. Counties list this organization in the telephone book in various ways: Aging, Council on Aging, or Department of Human Services. Long-distance caregivers can learn how to contact this agency in other states.

▸ Their introduction package may include comprehensive lists of day-care centers, in-home health care, and nursing facilities. These lists may include size, services provided, cost, and a thumbnail sketch of each center or facility.

▸ In Fairfax County, Virginia, the agency housed a long-term care ombudsman. The agency also arranged transportation to and from the day-care center and managed Meals on Wheels. A home companions' registry listed more than one hundred names from four counties, and included their experience, services provided, fees, and preferred hours.

Children of Aging Parents

This nonprofit organization provides help-line services, referrals, a network of support groups, publications, and programs promoting public awareness about the needs of caregivers. They should be especially useful for long-distance caregiving. Contact them at 800-227-7294, www.CAPS4caregivers.org or P.O. Box 167, Richboro, PA 18954.

Elder Care Locator (ELC)

ELC is a free referral service of the Administration on Aging, U.S. Department of Health and Human Services. ECL will contact the Area Agency on Aging in as many counties as needed. This is especially useful for long-distance caregiving. Services include data on care facilities in specific areas within a county and on special needs, such as Alzheimer's units or a small homelike situation. One may reach them at 800-677-1116 or go to www.aoa.gov and follow the links (Elder & Families, For Caregivers, Help-Where to find it).

Faith in Action

This is a national program of The Robert Wood Johnson Foundation with direction and technical assistance provided by the Wake Forest University School of Medicine. They have more than a thousand programs nationwide of interfaith volunteers, who provide non-nursing help. Help may include companionship, errands, phone calls, transportation, household tasks, and the loan of products. They could be especially good for long-distance caregiving. One can reach them at 877-324-8411 or www.faithinaction.org.

Family, immediate

One's family can provide exceptional support throughout all of the years. The type of support should adapt to the ever-changing circumstances. These are the ideas that worked in our family.

Independent Phase

The family dinners, cards, reciprocal visits, encouraging words, and empathy gave me great moral support. They also provided companionship for June.

The most depressing times for me were shortly before and after diagnosis. The most important role of our family was acting as a catalyst to get me started in my new role as caregiver. My son found a neuro-psychiatrist. My daughter obtained information about the Area Agency on Aging volunteer programs to give June constructive things to do. Both my daughter and mother-in-law motivated me to apply for Social Security Disability. My daughter found a live-in student nurse and partially completed the application for a day-care center.

Dependent and Final Phases

During these phases, my family provided most of my social activities. These included spending vacations, holidays, specials days, and sometimes just a relaxing day together.

One should limit how much caregiving for which one asks. Only ask for emergency help of three hours or less. For example, during one six-month period, my temporary loss of respite support caused me to ask for help about three times a month.

Internet

If someone does not have a computer, most public libraries have access to the Internet. Some allow reservations by phone (usually a half-hour). Arrive early to read the instruction manual. Although it may sound hard, it will be easier with experience (and the staff is always there to help).

When I first used a web browser, entering "Alzheimer's" as a keyword resulted in 952,000 sites. Search engines have improved dramatically since then. Nevertheless, getting a starter set of referrals is extremely helpful, so I have scattered references to sites throughout this book. One can then use these sites to research products and services.

Ombudsman

A long-term care ombudsman acts as an impartial third party in resolving problems. One can usually reach a county ombudsman through the county Area Agency on Aging. One gave me a four-page model agreement between employer and provider. Some nursing facilities have a volunteer ombudsman. These volunteers can help protect residents' rights, speak with the staff for those who cannot speak, and help with problems that residents cannot resolve alone.

The state of Virginia listed their ombudsman under Aging in the government section of the telephone book. When a nursing facility charged more than the amount prescribed, I asked for the drug dispensing records. The staff made excuses why they could not give the records and said there would be a significant charge involved if they did. The state ombudsman told me that I had a legal right to these records and the only possible charge should be for copying. Armed with this information, I obtained the records at no charge in eleven days and significantly reduced the drug charges.

Religion

When a doctor makes a diagnosis, share this information with the head of your local house of worship. That person can be a source of comfort and may help one counter depression. Some houses of worship now have a caregiver coordinator or parish nurse, who may help with other needs.

Finding a service at a time when one is free is not always easy. However, a retirement home in my area held a daytime communion service the second Thursday of every month. Ever more houses of worship have Saturday and Sunday evening services. People who do not practice a religion may find moral and spiritual support at a local Ethical Society.

Safe Return Program

The Alzheimer's Association sponsors this program that helps return a wanderer home safely. To get an information brochure, call 888-572-8566. The registration fee includes an easily recognizable lapel pin and bracelet. Both have the Alzheimer's Association logo on the front. The back of the bracelet says *Memory Impaired* along with a toll-free number and the family member's first name and ID. It is highly unlikely that someone with dementia can remove the bracelet. Caregivers give identifying information for a person with dementia, phone numbers of the local police, and three contacts. For a small additional fee, one may get a caregiver identification bracelet that alerts others that one provides care for a person registered in *Safe Return*. (Also see Wandering in the Tips chapter)

State Social Services Department

States sometimes have special programs or grants for caregivers. One is most likely to hear of these opportunities if one is a member of a support group and organizations involved with dementia.

Support group

The staff at the National Institute on Aging strongly recommended that I join a support group. To find the closest one, call the local Alzheimer's Association.

In our support group, I learned about a lawyer, training classes, arranging day care transportation, and where to go for overnight respite. Our group openly shared information and emotions.

Sample advice to new caregivers

Most new caregivers resisted the idea of respite care. An old-timer said, "If one kills oneself while caregiving, what alternative will there be for your family member? A period of challenge-free caregiving merely lulls one into a sense of complacency. When a new problem arises, it is usually too late to seek help."

Others resisted the use of prescription drugs. Old-timers told them both the benefits and side effects of drugs so they would have realistic expectations. The veterans also dispelled fears of inconti-

Notes

nence. New caregivers also learned not to worry about minor things, such as harmless behavioral changes. Support went beyond the group meetings. One call to my home lasted for ninety minutes.

Emotions

Newer caregivers sometimes felt the need to release their anger and guilt feelings. Everyone tried to be as supportive as possible. Most of all, everyone enjoyed a good laugh.

▸ President Bush visited the Alzheimer's wing of a long-term care facility. Smiling broadly, he stopped at a participant. He asked, "Do you know who I am?" The participant returned his smile and said "No, but if you go to the nurses' station, I'm sure someone there can tell you."

▸ An only child told her caregiving mother, "If you die before Dad, I'll kill you." (A true story)

LESSONS LEARNED

▸ Good moderators did not let a few persons dominate sessions, increased participation by asking questions, and redirected questions to experienced caregivers.

▸ A new caregiver should bring written questions as a reminder to every meeting.

▸ Mark the meeting dates on a calendar far in advance. (Caregivers can be forgetful.)

U.S. Department of Veterans Affairs

Any military veteran with a discharge other than dishonorable is eligible for a standard government grave monument. To apply, one must submit a VA Form 40-1330, which one may obtain from a cemetery or the U.S. Department of Veteran Affairs. Check a local phone book. If not listed, call 800-827-1000 (TTY 800-829-4833) or visit the web site at www.va.gov.

INTERNATIONAL RESOURCES

Alzheimer's Disease International (www.alz.co.uk/h associations.html)

This site lists Alzheimer's Associations around the world. It lists Europe and Latin America regional groups. Some countri lists are:

ALZHEIMER'S AUSTRALIA
P.O. Box 108
Higgins ACT 2615
Australia
Helpline: 1.800.639.331
www.alzheimers.org.au

ALZHEIMER SOCIETY of CANADA
20 Eglinton Avenue, W., Suite 1200
Toronto, Ontario M4R 1K8
Canada
Helpline: 1.800.616.8816
www.alzheimer.ca

ALZHEIMER SOCIETY
of IRELAND
Alzheimer's House
43 Northumberland Avenue
Dunlaoghaire, Co Dublin
Ireland
Helpline: 1.800.341.341
www.alzheimer.ie

ALZHEIMER'S NEW ZEALAND
Level 3, Adelphi Finance House
15 Courtenay Place
PO Box 3643
Wellington
New Zealand
Helpline: 0800.004.001
www.alzheimers.org.nz

ALZHEIMER SCOTLAND
ACTION on DEMENTIA
22 Drumsheugh Gardens
Edinburgh EH3 7RN
Scotland
Helpline: 0808.808.3000
www.alzscot.org

ALZHEIMER'S SOCIETY
(United Kingdom except Scotland)
Gordon House
10 Greencoat Place
London SW1P 1PH
United Kingdom
Helpline: 0845.300.0336
www.alzheimers.org.uk

Notes

Day-by-Day Living

June had been our family's chief caregiver. At first, my lack of skills left me at a disadvantage. Later, it became a blessing, because I had no preconceived ideas or habits to unlearn. That freedom allowed me to tailor caregiving to her needs.

Initially, family members can do all of the activities independently. These ideas can allow them to extend their independence and maintain their quality of life longer. When family members can only partially complete these activities, ideas in these chapters will allow them to maintain their dignity longer. Eventually, a family member will become totally dependent, and these activities will consume most of a caregiver's time. For this situation, one will learn simple solutions that can be done safely within the time available, while retaining respect for the family member.

Two factors greatly affect how well a family member can do these activities. An illness (some undetected) and prescription drugs both dramatically lower one's awareness. In the third year of the final phase, for example, my wife had fewer urinary tract infections and had stopped taking drugs. That helped her to relearn some activities even after her second seizure of the year.

Many right ways (and some wrong and even dangerous ways) of doing caregiving tasks exist. By trial and error, I found effective and simple solutions that worked for me. All these solutions may not, and should not, work for others. Instead, one should use those ideas appropriate to tailoring one's care.

Some information in these chapters now seems elementary. Nevertheless, it would have helped the novice that I was. I usually found others who could have benefited too. So I ask that more natural caregivers bear with the rest of us.

Chapter 11
Bathing

Companionship Phase

June bathed independently. Her modesty caused her to take tub baths behind closed doors, so learning exactly when challenges started was difficult.

Dependent Phase

In the first year, she could bathe with supervision. To maintain her skills and preserve her dignity, I only interjected a verbal prompt as necessary: "Here, dip the washcloth in the water. Now, rub this soap on the washcloth. Start washing your face."

In the second year, she needed extensive assistance. Getting her up from a sitting position became physically demanding. I could not do it without cooperation—sometimes slow in coming. I simulated a low grab bar with my arm. She could not concentrate, however, on simultaneously holding tight and lifting herself. As she lost the ability to help in getting herself out of the tub, bathing became my hardest daily task. In addition, various aspects of bathing were four of the eight things that I enjoyed the least. To avoid risking injury to us both, I started giving showers. By the third year, she totally depended on others for bathing.

Final Phase

The first two years, she stepped in and out of the tub, tried to get up from the transfer bench, and occasionally lifted a foot for me to wash. In the last two years, she still closed her eyes during a shampoo and rinsing, and held tightly onto a grab bar.

SHOWERS

After buying a few helpful products (e.g., a bath transfer bench) and developing better techniques, bathing became simpler. I tailored three showers to her situation: mini, standing, and sitting. All used a hand-held shower. I gave at least one every day.

Common solutions

▸ Keep the bathroom warm, which is important for someone whose homeostatic systems may function erratically.

▸ If family members stub a toe on the metal bathtub stopper, it will probably frighten them. Remove the stopper, or cover that area with a bathtub mat.

▸ Sometimes fidgeting or clutching the washcloth or hand-held shower interferes with the process. Try giving another wash-cloth for one hand and a tennis ball for the other hand. The best permanent solution is to install a grab bar. It satisfies the urge to hold. Because it is stationary, it also eliminates fidgeting.

▸ After incontinence begins, use a different colored washcloth for her face and upper body.

▸ Before starting, adjust the water to the right temperature and warm the washcloth. It may get confusing which side of the washcloth one soaps, so soap both sides.

▸ Since one will often have only one hand free, it helps having a smaller bar of soap. Use round bars or break a family size in half.

▸ Use either mild Ivory soap or unscented Dove. The former is easier to rinse, and the latter is kinder to the skin.

▸ Doing the shower without pause will decrease fidgeting.

▸ Use the hand-held shower only on its low (gentle) setting.

▸ To change positions, don't try to move her backwards (a prompt to sit). Instead, initiate a slow turn. Remind her to keep standing, and make sure that her hand firmly grips a grab bar.

▸ To prevent slips after a bath, keep a supply of paper towels by the tub. Dry the floor of the bathroom and the bathtub sides and top before she steps out. Keep a large non-slip area rug outside the tub for her to step out on.

Mini shower (:10, as needed)

Give a standing mini shower to clean areas that need attention. One should give it as a prelude to a sitting shower, but it may also be stand-alone.

▸ Rinse the appropriate areas with the hand-held shower. By hand, gently soap any sensitive or sore areas. Use a baby washcloth to soap other areas. One does not have to soap the entire body.

Standing shower (:20, from once to twice a week)—complete soaping, excluding a shampoo.

▸ The hand-held shower makes it possible for the caregiver to stand outside the tub. Keep the shower curtain partly closed to prevent water from coming out.

▸ Wash the closest parts of the body (usually her back).

▸ Turn your family member to wash the other side.

▸ Reduce the danger of falling by soaping feet last and rinsing them first. If one has trouble in raising a foot, skip the soap.

▸ Holding onto the grab bar is more important for your family member, so wash her hands later.

Sitting shower (:30, weekly—complete soaping and a shampoo.

▸ Before seating, warm the bench with water. Then dry it to prevent sliding.

▸ Shampoo—getting soap in an eye is less likely if one starts soaping hair from the back. The same idea applies for rinsing. As the water first starts to trickle onto the face, prompt her to close her eyes and quickly bring the water down over the front of the hair.

▸ Have her lean forwards while seated and hold the grab bar with one hand. Then gently pull her other arm forward to wash her back.

▸ When soaping eyes, move the washcloth down slowly from her forehead, while giving an oral prompt. This should cause her eyes to close. Sometimes a family member will open her eyes immediately after soaping, so rinse them first. Start slowly rinsing above the forehead. Simultaneously, shield her eyes with one hand. An oral prompt and the trickle of water will cause her eyes to close. (Also rinse any soap off the bench to prevent her from sliding off.)

▸ To avoid getting water in her ears, one should cup a hand around an ear and aim the water above the ear. Use a finger to flick out the ear afterwards.

▸ Wash feet last. To avoid tipping her backward, barely raise each foot.

DRYING

▸ To prevent prematurely exiting from a tub, make sure her hands stay on the grab bar.

▸ Use one towel for the upper body and another for the waist down.

▸ While in the tub, only dry those parts of the body that cannot be dried while sitting.

▸ Exit the tub and dry the remaining parts while seated on the toilet. Allow a few minutes of airing out time.

Use a blow dryer for rashes

▸ Before using a blow dryer on your family member, try it on yourself to learn the best settings (e.g., the blower on high and heat on low) and distance. With handle controls, avoid accidentally flipping the heat setting from low to high.

▸ Check the less obvious areas (the groin and between the toes) for rashes. Even after one cures a rash, continue using the blow dryer as a preventive measure.

▸ While drying the feet, one should inspect (visually and by feel) them for other problems. Let the air from the dryer bounce off your cupped hand to dry the soles.

▸ To dry the area between the legs completely, one must stand. To prevent accidents, keep a fitted brief between her legs to make it easier to pull up quickly.

BED BATH

Getting to a bathtub may be temporarily difficult or impossible. Bed baths served us well until I installed a stair lift that allowed us to use the upstairs bath again.

▸ To prepare for a bed bath, cut a piece of plastic to overlap the hospital bed by a foot on all sides. Keep handy two beach towels, several other towels, three plastic washbasins and four washcloths. (As Winston Churchill said "Nothing succeeds like excess.") Towels also help to soak up excess water. Pull a table close for the basins—one with soapy water and two with rinse water. Use hot water because it cools quickly. Use mild Ivory soap.

▸ After helping a family member to stand, cover the bed with plastic and put a beach towel over the plastic. After helping her undress, provide normal incontinence care. Place her on her back and cover her with the second beach towel. Raise the side rails.

▸ To ease bending, raise the hospital bed to its maximum height.

▸ Raise the head of the bed to its maximum height. Wring most of the soap out of the washcloth and quickly wash the face. To wash the eyes, merely wipe once from the nose outward.

▸ Lower the head of the bed to wash the rest of the body. Work from the top down, uncovering only the part being washed.

▸ Then roll her onto a side and wash her backside.

▸ To avoid leaving a soap residue (and causing a rash), use a double rinse with fresh hot water before drying.

Chapter 12
Dressing/Undressing

SITUATIONS BY PHASE

Companionship phase

June dressed independently, but a few challenges appeared early. By the last year, dressing required supervision.

Confusion

▶ Give away those clothes that a person does not wear. Store out-of-season clothes in spare closets. In the primary closet, separate tops and bottoms and group them by color. To make smaller things easy to find, clear a large upper dresser drawer for a one-stop shopping location for socks, stockings, panties, and bras. Label each drawer and closet appropriately.

Frustration in choosing outfits

▶ Offer a limited choice of matching items.
▶ Buy new clothes in matching colors.

Increased frustration in choosing outfits

▶ Lay out a color-coordinated outfit in the order to be put on.
▶ If the order becomes mixed up, hand each item in the correct order.

Dependent phase

During the first two years, dressing required extensive assistance. Later in this phase, dressing required total assistance, but she still raised her feet to put them into her pants.

Resistance to dressing or undressing

▸ Before trying any other solution, saying, "You can help" sometimes overcomes the resistance and may cause cooperation.

Difficulty in putting on pants due to constant motion

▸ Have a comfortable place to sit in the dressing area.

Final phase

During this phase, she sometimes pulled an undershirt down and lifted her feet to take her pants off. At first, she stuck her arms into sleeves. Later, she occasionally raised an arm to put into a sleeve, but did not uncurl her hand to ease going through them. Even in the last year, she held her feet still while I put on her socks and helped occasionally to pull tops on or off.

Excessive laundry

▸ Clothes usually get soiled after breakfast. Use outer clothes from the night before until bath time.

DRESSING SITUATIONS

Maintaining skills

▸ Dress in the same sequence. If one always starts with the same arm, she may help by raising it. Following a bath, put her brassiere or undershirt on slowly so she can help. Do not pull it down. Modesty will usually cause that to happen. Allow lots of time. A person will find it easier to put on an undershirt. When putting on an over-the-head garment, spread the sleeve opening with one's fingers. Then hold the opening where a family member may easily put in an arm.

The fright of having an over-the-head garment temporarily blocking vision

▸ After seating for safety, gather the entire garment in both hands, with the head opening free. Approach with the head opening in front to avoid impairing vision. Then rotate the rest of the garment back and over the head.

The garment is long (e.g., a nightgown) or she slumps against the back of the bench

▸ Get the arms in and wait until standing to pull the item down.

Spreading fingers while inserting a hand into a sleeve, or clutching the sleeve
▸ Ask gently for cooperation. If she does not give it, reach in from the bottom of the sleeve and pull her hand through.

The hand not going into a sleeve holds the sleeve shut
▸ To give that hand something else to hold, wrap it around your forearm.

Too much foot motion to put on socks and shoes
▸ Sit on one's haunches (or a stool) and put one foot between one's knees, with her leg straight. Draping an outstretched leg across the top of one's thigh is also effective.

Putting on very tight surgical hose (to counteract leg swelling)
▸ The large *V* shaded part of the hose top must be in the front. Then sprinkle baby powder on one's hand and rub your family member's feet until they are slippery.

Trying to put a heel first into a pant leg may tear off a toenail.
▸ Putting socks on first protects nails. Start socks, pants, and shoes on whatever foot she raises first. Reach up the pant leg to point the toe. That should prompt pushing the foot through. If not, gently pull the foot through.

Putting both feet in the same pant leg
▸ Start seated. With one hand between the pants legs and the other hand on the rear top of the pants, guide the pants up.

To avoid the exertion of getting up an extra time
▸ With her pants only partly on, put her shoes on.

An imbalance after standing
▸ Stand still for a few moments until she no longer needs support.

Maintaining the skill of putting on pants
▸ After standing, wait to see if she will pull up her pants without help.

An imbalance caused by your trying to tuck in a shirt/blouse while pulling pants up
▸ After a skirt or pants are all the way up, reseat to tuck in the shirt or blouse.

Blouse sleeves jamming high on arms when putting a sweater over a top
  ‣ Reach through the sweater sleeve from the cuff, hold onto the cuff of the blouse, and then guide the arm through the sweater sleeve.

Fidgeting while standing
  ‣ Reseat her for zipping a jacket.
  ‣ If the garment has Velcro, don't bother using any other fasteners.

UNDRESSING SITUATIONS

Loss of mental ability to pull arms out of sleeves when taking off a coat
  ‣ After unfastening, take the coat by the collar and peel the top half back and down. Then, one at a time, the sleeves slip off easily. Since this takes two hands, however, ensure family members have something soft (sofa) behind them in case of loss of balance.

Fidgeting while unbuttoning shirts/blouses
  ‣ For safety, seat before unbuttoning.

Maintaining skills
  ‣ For tops, ask her to raise her arms. Then take off both top and undershirt simultaneously so she does not have to raise arms twice.

Taking off tops when she tightly clenches the sleeve cuff
  ‣ Start with, "Good job, thank you." If she resists, hold hands and slide the sleeves unto your own arm. One may also stand behind, reach in from the top of the sleeve, and slowly *walk* a hand down the arm until the tightly clenched fingers relax.

Interference with taking off an undershirt
  ‣ Give her something to hold to keep her hands occupied.

To avoid the exertion of getting up an extra time
  ‣ Before seating, slip the pants below the hips.

Lifting a family member's heavy foot with your injured arm
- ▸ Slide a forearm under one of her thighs and rest that hand on top of the other thigh. Lifting then requires little effort.

Taking an over-the-head nightgown off while prone in bed
- ▸ Raise the front of the nightgown above the waist. Lift both legs and slide the back of the nightgown above the waist. After assisting to a sitting position, remove the gown.

Chapter 13
Eating

Through Companionship Phase
June ate independently. The only challenge was preventing over-eating.

Dependent Phase
The first year, June ate independently, but needed help to cut up food. During the next two years, she needed assistance, especially with soup. By the fourth year, she had trouble keeping a spoon upright. She needed extensive assistance, especially when tired (usually at dinner). By the last year, she could still spear and eat food with a fork, but no longer spat out an occasional seed. She dropped food often.

Final Phase
For the first two years, she could still eat with a fork if I helped her spear the pieces. Once, she even adjusted her fork into three different positions before she found one that allowed her to eat. Also, she didn't stick her tongue with a fork, as others occasionally did. She ate finger foods after I put them into her hand. On her best day, however, she picked up food, took a bite, and then set it back down. Glasses spilled when she forgot to set them down. Also, she did not voluntarily drink as much and began forgetting to swallow.

By the third year, she became almost totally dependent. On her best days, however, she fed herself hand-held foods if they were placed in her hand. She anticipated food and drink by opening her mouth without prompting and could hold a glass long enough to take the first sip. She swallowed more slowly and ate the last part of dinners with her eyes closed.

By the last year, she became totally dependent. She ate well at breakfast and lunch. By dinnertime, she started falling asleep and seldom ate more than a salad and part of the side dish or entree.

Appetite

One should worry about a slight change in appetite only if it lasts for more than one day. (Sometimes, a person has a slow day.)

Some causes of a decrease in appetite
▶ Changes in eating routines, exercise, liquids, or drugs
▶ Discomfort following return from a nursing facility—consider asking your doctor to check for a urinary tract infection.

Things to review
▶ General attitude and strength
▶ Possible problems of the teeth, gums and mouth
▶ Recent bowel habits (frequency and consistency)
▶ External signs (temperature, blood pressure, pulse)

Maintaining a good appetite
▶ If one finds food mouth-watering, a family member is apt to like it too. An "Um-m-m" reaction cannot be beat.
▶ Serve a person soup and other moist foods daily.
▶ Food should be easy to chew. Avoid food like toasted cheese sandwiches and caramels.
▶ Ambience and warmth help. Share meals with soft music, and hold hands if possible.
▶ In the later years, shift to more easily chewable food (cooked rather than raw vegetables).

Eating

Self-feeding preserves a family member's dignity and saves time for a caregiver. Reduce stress by not scheduling anything shortly after a meal. Serving one item at a time allows better concentration. If the bottom of a bowl or plate feels hot, it is too hot to eat. Throughout a meal, continually tell what is about to happen, even when one leaves the room.

Placement of dishes and utensils
▶ One should place dishes and utensils far enough back from the edge of the table so a family member is more likely to see them—usually about six inches. At that distance, she will feed herself more readily. It is also less likely that arms and sleeves will go into the food.
▶ Set out only one utensil—either a spoon or a fork. For the first mouthful, place a spoon under the food or spear the first item with a fork.

Prompts for self-feeding

Wait after each of these prompts to see if it causes self-feeding.

▸ Eat a first bite to show how tasty it is. Then, offer a small bite.

▸ Help your family member grasp the utensil close to the food, because she will usually move her hand (not the food) to her mouth.

▸ Slowly guide the full utensil into her mouth.

▸ After she swallows, slowly guide the utensil back to the food to refill it.

▸ If she stops in mid-meal, merely saying, "Eat your food" may restart self-feeding.

▸ If arms stiffen and are hard to bend to the plate, raise the plate to the hands.

Self-feeding with a spoon (almost through the dependent phase)

As drugs peak, your family member may have difficulty holding a spoon without spilling its contents.

▸ Larger spoons may enable her to get a partial spoonful.

▸ Switch to bite-sized foods.

▸ Feed the liquid part of soup and cereals first, so spooning the rest will be easier for her.

▸ Sometimes, the mouth does not close before she withdraws the spoon. Place the tip of your finger in front of the food so it will stay in her mouth as she withdraws the spoon. Plan to help more toward the end of a meal.

Self-feeding with a fork (through half the final phase)

▸ A person can more easily hold a fork if the thumb is on the opposite side from the other fingers.

▸ Using the fork as a spear is easier if the fork is placed into the hand upside down. Since the food may fall off otherwise, help to impale items securely.

▸ Start with the largest piece first. A person adapts more readily to increasingly smaller pieces.

▸ To avoid potential injury from an empty fork, keep a piece of food on the end of the fork and take the fork away after the last bite.

Hand-held foods

▸ If a family member has a preferred eating hand, place food where picking it up is most visible and convenient.

▸ Make portions easy to handle (e.g., cut sandwiches in half or quarters).

▸ Fold any messy food (e.g., toast and jam), in half. Keep a wet cloth handy for messy hands.

▸ As more food goes on the floor, do not make food available until she swallows the previous piece. Then place food securely into a hand. If this does not start self-feeding, guide a hand until the food touches the lips. If one sees an arm stretch out to drop food, say, "That is yours. Keep it."

Feeding with a spoon

To avoid accidentally piercing a tongue with a fork, feed with a spoon.

▸ A family member will seldom open wide for the first spoonful, so use a small amount.

▸ Keeping the spoon visible, slowly move it toward the mouth (a prompt to open). Touching the spoon to the upper lip will also usually cause the mouth to open. (The lower lip may not work as well. If the mouth suddenly opens with force, it may spill the food or even knock the spoon out of your hand.)

▸ Sometimes, she may not open her mouth, but will only suck food off the tip of the spoon. Choking could occur, so pause before retrying feeding.

▸ Liquids—put a spoon in soup well in advance and give the first spoonful empty to make sure that the soup is not too hot. Keeping a spoon level is easier if one is standing. To avoid dripping, do not fill the spoon. On a day with lots of spillage, move the bowl under the chin.

▸ Have patience (count to ten between spoonfuls).

Challenges in the early phases

▸ Sometimes, a family member reluctantly relinquishes utensils or crockery, saying, "No, it's mine." Consider trading that utensil for another used in the next course. Also consider saying, "Good Job" and "Thank you," while taking the utensil.

▸ Drug side effects cause slow eating. To while away the time, eat your meals simultaneously. Sit close enough to feed, but far enough away to safeguard your food.

▸ Stop if she clamps her teeth on a utensil. When she relaxes, take the utensil out rather than in. Pause before restarting.

▸ Reactions respond to actions. For example, if one quickly lowers a family member's hand to spear food, expect a quick jerking back, which could result in an injury.

▸ Sometimes, one may feel as if running a gauntlet of hands (one of her hands may even interfere with self-feeding). Slowly lower hands and stroke them until they relax. Consider holding hands. If the hands are too active, take a short pause. (She may only want to scratch an ear.) Also, consider keeping hands busy by curling them around the edge of the geriatric chair tray.

Challenges in the later phases

▶ To avoid having them knocked to the floor, keep plates and bowls far out of harms way.

▶ Chewing meat took a long time, but chewing a large piece took no longer than a small one. One can feed an entire rectangular piece if one puts it in sideways (rather than end first).

▶ To avoid rushing, relax your head on her shoulder (to hear when chewing finishes).

▶ For safety, do not leave a family member alone during a meal. To prevent her head from lolling back (and causing her to choke), either cradle it in your arm or support it with a pillow. As swallowing takes place, immediately give another spoonful.

▶ If chewing or swallowing stops, touch a lip with an empty spoon. That should trigger vigorous chewing and swallowing. When one senses the end of eating, massage the jaw muscles to prompt swallowing, and then clear the mouth with your finger.

Food buying

Shortly after I became a full-time caregiver, the Washington Post ran an article by Nina Killham called *A Commonsense Guide to Storing Foods*. She said, "Toss the 4-year-old leftovers." After an inventory of refrigerator, pantry, and cabinets, I tossed everything I could not remember buying or did not remember using. I tossed seven opened cornstarch boxes and got rid of most herbs and spices. The shelves on the door of the refrigerator emptied quickly.

After that, I bought a different quantity or size. If we did not consume an item within two weeks, I bought smaller sizes (e.g., condiments and eggs) and switched to six-packs of most juices. For foods we ate frequently, I paid a lower price by buying larger sizes.

Buy continence-friendly food

▶ One hundred percent whole wheat breads provide the most fiber.

▶ We ate cereals with high dietary fiber, low total fat, and no saturated or trans fats. *Extra Fiber* All-Bran (15-1-0), Fiber

One (13-1-0), and All-Bran (10-2-0) best satisfied our criteria. Since these numbers may change, check the *Nutrition Facts* on the side of the box.

▸ Lots of fruits and vegetables: One also does not have to cook some food (e.g., broccoli, carrots, cauliflower, celery, cucumbers, mushrooms, and peppers).

▸ Having soup once or twice a day also adds to one's liquid intake.

▸ Olive oil can replace butter/oleo and reduce total cholesterol without lowering HDL. By mixing it with various types of vinegar (e.g., balsamic), one can create very tasty salad dressings.

Other food to consider

▸ Anything that one can eat or assemble as hand-held food

▸ Vegetables (e.g., beans, corn, and potatoes) that one can add to meals cooked in large quantities

▸ Healthier desserts (e.g., graham crackers, frozen yogurt or low-fat ice cream)—avoid those with fruit or nuts; as awareness declines, the inconsistency becomes confusing.

▸ Fat-free milk and Lite Salt (it only has 50% sodium chloride)

▸ On the other hand, avoid caffeine to allow your family a good night's sleep.

Other considerations

▸ To maintain skills at each meal, plan about three items that may be easily self-fed. Breakfast: citrus, toast, and a banana. Lunch: sandwiches, fruit, and graham crackers. Dinner: carrots, bread, and sometimes fish sticks.

▸ To make weekends easier, have a microwave dinner.

▸ Keep extra supplies on hand for winter emergencies (e.g., tuna with noodles, pasta with meat sauce, soups, dehydrated milk, citrus, canned meats, and canned or dried fruits). Macaroni & Cheese always reminded me of the meatless nights during the early years of our marriage.

▸ To buy one's complete needs, keep a future-shopping list handy for updating. (One cannot easily run out *for* something when one runs out *of* something.)

Food preparation

Early phases

A family member feels good contributing to a meal (e.g., preparing salad and setting and clearing the table). After a family member forgets which utensils to set, just hand the correct ones to her.

Later phases

A family member is less likely to become agitated if a meal flows continuously (no wait times). One can achieve this with simple foods, prepared in advance.

▸ Breakfast—only serve cold meals weekdays (under the pressure of preparing for a bus pickup). Peel oranges (Temples were the easiest). To avoid cracked teeth, hold the pieces of citrus up to the natural light from a window to spot any hidden seeds. Arrange the pieces for easy spearing. Put milk on cereal early to soften it. Choking is less likely with less contrast between the solids and liquids.

▸ Dinner—precook enough food for many meals and freeze them in single meal containers. (See Appendix C for two easy ones.) These meals only need heating, so they allow one to spend more energy on a family member.

▸ Dinners-from-scratch—mine included very large (an eight-inch bowl) salads with lots of vegetables. I sliced the salad into easily spooned portions and mixed the salad dressing in well. Cooking potatoes or yams in the microwave took no more than ten minutes, and they stayed moist. One can easily chew carrots after one minute in the microwave (high setting).

▸ To warm frozen yogurt, set the microwave at half power for 1:30. It melts but is still cool.

▸ If one serves look-a-like food (e.g., two types of milk), use contrasting containers for each of you. (One may become confused after bringing identical glasses to the table.)

▸ During the years of slow self-feeding, one can prepare some items after the meal starts.

Meal routines

Prepare the largest quantity of food for the time of greatest alertness—usually breakfast. Talking (even if one-sided) during meals helps to pass the time and keeps one from becoming impatient if a family member chews slowly. The following routines worked for us in the later phases.

Meal locations

▸ We ate breakfast and lunch in our traditional manner—side-by-side at our kitchen table. We ate dinner in the family room so we could watch music videos too.

▸ After her hip replacement, June sat on the bath transfer bench on a plastic carpet runner next to her bed, with our trays on her bed.

Breakfast

To distract her while I put her bib on, I gave her the first slice of orange. We ate the rest of the meal simultaneously. While she finished her banana, I cleared the dishes.

Lunch

Because I stood to feed her soup, eating soup simultaneously was unnatural. So I ate my soup in the kitchen while she watched music videos in the family room. This also allowed me to relax for a short time. After I fed soup to her, we ate the remaining courses simultaneously. It took a long time for her to drink liquids, so she had sips throughput the meal.

Dinner

I fed salads (that took a long time to eat) while I slowly sipped wine. This kept me from rushing her and allowed both of us to finish the rest of the meal simultaneously.

Laughter was contagious

Midway through the dependent phase, June had her left elbow on the geriatric chair tray, with her arm straight up. Her outfit had a large sleeve, which stood open. She meticulously picked up the left-over dinner food with her other hand and carefully dropped each piece down her sleeve.

Chapter 14

Continence and Incontinence

Maintaining continence

Helping family members use the toilet preserves their dignity and reduces urinary tract infections. Although maintaining continence is the most important of the day-by-day living activities, it is also the most difficult to achieve. One may, however, achieve a goal of maintaining continence three-fourths of the time. Success can result from doing these things.

▶ Under doctor supervision, reduce drugs whenever possible.

▶ Eat the same foods to understand how your family member may respond to them.

▶ Achieving regularity and predictability will be more likely if one provides continence-friendly food and gives lots of liquids.

▶ Help a person to the toilet at least four times daily. Pick those times most likely to produce results (e.g., upon arising, midmorning before a bath, and just before bedtime).

▶ Urination frequently triggers a bowel movement. To trigger urination, give a drink of water after seating on the toilet. Running water in the sink or tub may also act as a trigger.

▶ Allow a person to have complete privacy and enough time (about fifteen minutes).

Other tips

When using a toilet safety frame, relax your family member against the back before leaving. To prevent arms getting wedged, make sure they are on the top or outside the metal frame arms. Use baby wipes after each use of the toilet, even if no apparent need exists (urinary tract infections occur easily).

Do not be discouraged by months/years of failure. Persistence pays off. (Even after three years, my wife successfully regained skills.)

Changing area

Of the activities of daily living, one has the least control over incontinence. The start of incontinence, however, will resolve the challenge resulting from a family member using the toilet, but not remaining seated long enough to complete the act. Prepare for this event at the beginning of the dependent phase. Set up a changing area with lots of room, including space to store extra supplies. (A double vanity sink works well.) Have a comfortable place for your family member to sit. Lay a plastic runner over the rug.

Keep supplies that one uses frequently in the handiest place. (One may want briefs, inserts, baby wipes, body lotion, disposable gloves, bandages, rash ointment, antibiotic, and a clock on the vanity top.) Prepare supplies for ready use (e.g., open the baby wipes' container). After your family member is no longer mobile, unscrew tops. Clear out the vanity cabinets for extra supplies. (One will appreciate having them within easy reach.)

Once mobility becomes a challenge, one may want a mini changing area on each floor. One only needs to keep briefs, wipes, disposable gloves, and a chair in a secondary area.

Changing briefs (underpants)

To preserve the dignity of your family member, call them underpants when talking to her.

Preparation

▸ A family member's fingers can be lethal weapons, so protect your eyes.

▸ Wear at least one disposable glove.

▸ For open-sided briefs, fasten one end of each strap—with the button on the outside. Add absorbent inserts to briefs at bedtime. To avoid putting on a brief backwards when rushed, lay it out the same way each time.

▸ To help your family member maintain better balance (and stand still long enough for one to finish changing a brief), adapt the following methods to her strength. If she can stand, find something solid that she can hold. (We used an area wall divider.) A doorknob may be enough to hold with one hand; push your foot against the door to keep it from moving. She can place the other hand on your neck or shoulder. (Make sure that it's not your ears or hair). Without a suitable support, lean your family member forward slightly with both hands on the wall. (This also keeps the hands from interfering with the process.) As physical deterioration takes place, a walker can help a family member stand.

Taking off a brief

As one takes off a fitted brief, refasten the straps. Otherwise, they will stick to anything and complicate removal.

Putting on a brief

▸ When one sits facing a side, centering a fitted brief front-to-back will be much easier. Pull the brief up so the top straps are above the waist. Fasten the two top straps first, starting with the closest one. Pulling the strap and the brief in opposite directions will give a snug fit. To keep the brief from being too snug, make sure that your finger can easily slip in the top and bottom. Before fastening the last top strap, pull the brief up again. After fastening each strap, run a finger over them to ensure secure sticking.

▸ As balance becomes poor, slip the brief between her legs while she is standing and then seat her to fasten the straps.

▸ Keep the brief dry or the straps will not stick.

▸ Omit the middle strap. When one takes the brief off and rolls them up, the unused strap will hold them together. This also lets more air get to the skin.

▸ If a person is bed-bound, consider not fastening the straps. This allows even more airing.

Preventing accidents

▸ Use fitted briefs exclusively. Check throughout the day to make sure its straps are secure, especially the bottom ones.

▸ Keep an absorbent underpad on the seat of the wheelchair, geriatric chair, other sitting areas, and the bed. (The underpad also provides warmth.)

Chapter 15

Moving from Place to Place

One may want to skip reading this chapter until dementia compromises a family member's movement. Then, one will find that the detail will answer some important questions. Before trying some of these techniques, however, one should evaluate one's strength versus the weight of one's family member.

June's weight peaked at 165 pounds at the end of the companionship phase and again at 162 pounds in the second year of the final phase. She had unsteady legs but great upper body strength. We moved from place to place a minimum of twenty-one times each day. Under those conditions, improperly transferring from one position or place to another could have resulted in debilitating accidents.

LESSONS LEARNED

Some safety precautions are common to all movement.

▸ Allow a person lots of time to avoid moving at an unsafe speed. Going at the pace of your family member should achieve this. Moving slowly also allows one the time to react at the first sign of one's own pain.

▸ Anticipate complications and take precautions against them. For example, to keep a person's hands from interfering during a difficult movement, put one of her arms around your shoulder and reach behind her back to hold the other.

▸ To prevent self-injuries, replace strength with leverage and skill. Stand or kneel close to your family member to decrease having to bend or stretch. Your feet or knees should be shoulder-width apart. Point yourself in the direction that your family member needs to move. Bend knees (rather than one's back), or squat to use stronger leg muscles. Use two arms to lighten loads and rest the greatest weight closer to your elbows.

Automobile

In case of an accident getting into a car, open the garage to make a call for help easier. June could not get over the threshold in our garage, so I pushed her geriatric chair up to the sill. When I helped her out, her feet came down on the far side of the sill. As one goes past the car door, open it slightly because one cannot reach the door handle later without letting go of one's family member. As one opens the car door wider, stand far enough away so the door will clear her. Hold the upper corner to prevent it hitting her. To prevent a person from clinging to a part of the car, hold both of her hands in one of yours. Keep one hand behind her head to keep it from hitting the car. Prompt her to sit and ease her left arm and shoulder into the car. As she sits, push her hips in as far as possible with your left knee.

Then step into the car with your right foot, tuck her arms in, pick up her feet, and swing them into the car. Her body will naturally follow. Use your right knee to guide her back so she will have plenty of knee room. To avoid getting her hand or arm pinched, slowly close the door within an inch before slamming it.

If one gets out next to a curb, pull the two tires on her side onto the curb to make it easier to get out. Then turn the motor off, unlock her door, and shift into a gear. (Once, she almost released the emergency brake while I walked to her side of the car.) To exit, lift her feet and swing them out. Her body follows naturally. To avoid hitting her head, prompt her to duck her head. If she does not, keep a hand between her head and the car. Holding one or preferably both hands, lift her to her feet.

Bathtub

Getting into the tub

Wearing a pair of beach thongs should prevent your slipping accidentally. The challenge of getting into the tub resembled the ride of a steeplechase jockey. The slightest hesitation or lack of confidence on my part caused us to fail. By approaching without pause, we succeeded 80% of the time. If she did not step in, we backed up and tried several more times until we succeeded.

For a short time following her hip replacement, we used the transfer bench to enter the tub. The seat extended far enough out of the tub so one may sit before sliding over. Then we rotated her legs in. To get out, one reverses that procedure.

Getting out of the tub

During the first two years of the final phase, June regularly got out with only verbal cues from me. In the third year, she needed some assistance. In her last year, she occasionally stepped in or out of the tub without prompting. With prompting, she did it more frequently, but usually needed help in lifting the first leg.

For safety and balance, one should step into the tub with one foot and spread one's feet wide. Place an arm around your shoulder. While holding onto the grab bar, transfer her other arm from the grab bar to oneself. Then do a dance-like turn until she faces out. Your arm holding the grab bar will be against her back and give her a feeling of security. Use a prompt to get her to step out. Even if she raises a leg only slightly, it reduces the physical strain of lifting that leg over the side. Her second leg will follow.

Bed

Going to bed

In the second year of the dependent phase, June could still put herself to bed, but wound up awkwardly splayed across the bed. To position her comfortably, I knelt on the bed with my knees where I wanted her to be. Then I leaned back and let my body weight move her. (My body and shoulders did the pulling, not my arms.)

By the following year, she could seldom scoot herself onto the bed and needed extensive assistance to position herself comfortably. Use prompts in this situation to get your family member to sit at the midpoint of the bed and scoot up on the bed. Be patient and allow extra time to do that. If unsuccessful, stand as close to the bed as possible, keeping your back straight and knees bent. Then put the crook of one arm under her knees and the other arm slanted across her back to her armpit. Using her bottom as a pivot point, rotate her on the bed to help her lie down.

Getting up

Prop up both her knees and put both of your forearms under them. Lifting only the knees, rotate her body. With her legs hanging over the side, hold her arms and raise her to a standing position.

Geriatric chair

In the winter, store the chair near a hot air register so the metal parts may warm. The tray and footrest slide more easily if one occasionally wipes the inner metal tubes with a damp cloth and dries them. The chair has hard-to-use brakes. So back the chair near a wall in case it rolls. As one nears the chair, turn her around and release her hand closest to the chair. (That way, she will more readily reach back to grab an arm of the chair.) Steady the chair and pause to give her a chance to grab both arms and scoot herself into a comfortable position. If not, then slowly put your arms under her arms and clasp your hands in front of her. A prompt should cause her to put her feet on the footrest. Another prompt should cause her to push back as one gives a gentle backward tug to get her all the way back.

One must retract the footrest to make it easy for her to seat herself. For her to rest her feet comfortably, however, one must pull it back out. By bracing one's shoulders against the chair and one's forearms against one's thighs, the leverage gained will allow one to pull the footrest partially out with two hands easily. (I hurt an arm doing it one-handed.) Place her feet on the footrest before pulling it out all the way. When putting the tray up, keep one hand between it and her stomach. That way, one can make sure it is not too snug.

Occasionally, one may want to move the chair with a family member in it. To prevent fright, stop before thresholds and say, "Here's a bump," and go over it slowly. To avoid injury, go slowly through doorways because viselike hands may often grip both sides.

Sometimes, a family member prevents one from removing the tray and letting her out. Since one raises the tray from left to right, slowly remove her left hand and raise the tray past it before moving her other hand. Then wait a moment to encourage her to get up by herself.

One should push the footrest in before removing the tray. (Getting out of the chair quickly once, she tipped it over by putting all her weight on the footrest.) To push the footrest back, I had to lift her feet. After an arm injury, I did not have enough strength to lift them. In a crouched position, I rested my left forearm on my left thigh and lifted her legs with my left arm. The leverage made it easy. Simultaneously, I pushed the footrest back with my right arm. To avoid straining my fingers, I pushed with the meaty part of the palm.

Sitting/Getting up

Sitting

June eventually sat with more force. Once, another caregiver backed her up (a cue to sit), and she scraped her back as she slid past the front of a wooden seat to the floor. To avoid that, approach from the side until your family member is next to a sitting area. Then she only has to make a quarter-turn to be in the right position. Before she sits, guide one of her hands to an armrest. (If she ever sat alone, I hoped she would reach back by habit.) After she grips the armrest, release her second hand. That should cause her to use more of her own effort to sit. If the sitting area does not have an armrest, simulate one with your arm. Once seated, a pillow on each side will keep her upright. Disposable absorbent under pads in the sitting areas allows sitting without concern.

Since space around a toilet is cramped, walk in together and brace yourself against a wall with feet spread wide. Then slowly lower your family member to the hard seat.

Getting up from the floor

Before doing this movement, one should evaluate the risk. To get a family member up from the floor, help her sit with her knees drawn up. With one foot wedged directly in front of both of hers, lean back to allow your body weight to help raise her.

Getting up from furniture with an arm

Hold one arm and put her other hand on the furniture arm. Gently nudge upward on the arm to prompt her to push herself up using her own strength. If she is too weak, prompt her to scoot forward. One foot in front of hers should prevent her from sliding to the floor. Then place one of her hands around your waist to maintain her balance and her other hand around your arm. One should space one's feet far apart to maintain balance. After she is up, pause to make sure that she has her balance.

STAIRS

We had to traverse stairs because our living and sleeping/bathing rooms were on separate floors. It became physically difficult and time-consuming for me, but excellent exercise for my wife. Through the companionship years, June handled stairs alone. For the first three years of the dependent phase, I merely watched to guard against accidents. By the next year, I had to take an active role.

Originally, I only gave cursory coverage to stairs. In the fourth year of the dependent phase, however, a very experienced home companion and her nurse supervisor struggled for about an hour before calling 911 for assistance. Since this task normally took about one minute, I realized that others might not know some simple techniques. Even worse, I became concerned that other caregivers might be doing something too risky. The following techniques avoided injury in more than six years. It may seem like much detail, but these details may prevent accidents.

Initially, I found it easier to position myself in front. As her balance worsened in the second year of the final phase, I tailored my position based on the situation.

‣ Well-lit stairs increase safety and cooperation.
‣ On approaching stairs, release the hand closest to the banister to encourage your family member to reach for it. If not, place her hand on it. Do not move until her hand grips it. The banister helps to maintain balance and prevents staggers. One should also tightly grip the banister and wrap one's fingers around the back of an upright support.
‣ Unless it can drape over your arm, don't carry anything.
‣ Watch her feet and her hand on the banister to see when she is ready for the next step. When either moves, it is an indicator that she is ready to move.
‣ For a short time after hip surgery, one may need to give a gentle encouraging tug.
‣ Prompts and encouraging words are extremely important ("Lift your leg" or, "You are doing a good job"). As one nears the end, say, "Just a few more steps." When she looks as though she needs a pause, stop prompting. After she traversed all the steps in either direction, I said, "Good job."

Stairs (down only)

Dependent Phase

Going down took twice the time as going up—about two minutes in total, but up to fifteen seconds for each first and last step.

‣ To avoid her accidentally bumping me down before I braced myself, I stayed far back on the stair landing. Only then did I bring her to the landing. After getting a firm grip with one hand, I positioned myself.
‣ The first step took the most time. I waited for her to inch her way slowly up to it.
‣ As an additional precaution against falls, I braced myself several steps below and leaned toward her.
‣ So I could watch both her feet and her hand on the rail, I focused my eyes halfway between them and used my peripheral vision.
‣ For safety, I exerted gentle pressure only after she started to step. Then I gently placed a hand on the back of a foot until it cleared the previous step.
‣ She often led with the same foot. So that she would use the other foot as well, I turned her body on the last step so she

would use the less-used foot. I encouraged her with, "Use your other foot."

▶ She came close to tripping only on the last step. I had relaxed, so I learned to concentrate until the end.

Final Phase

As she slowed, the act of stepping had three distinct parts with a pause between each: preparation, stepping down, and completion. Timing of encouraging words helped. Understanding these phases enabled me to help her descend in about five minutes.

In the preparation phase, she shuffled up to the edge of the step. I prompted her with, "Ready?" If she hesitated, I said, "You are doing very well." As she started to reach out hesitantly with a foot, I said, "That's it" (sometimes more than once). That caused her to continue instead of pulling her foot back.

In the next phase, she stepped down. For encouragement, I said, "Step down." I anticipated a possible loss of balance. As she prepared to move a foot, I leaned my head near her stomach and braced my forearm on top of the banister rail. When I saw foot movement, I said, "Here we go," and I backed down. That motivated her to continue stepping down. If she took her hand off the banister, I replaced it lower so she had to bend her knees slightly to reach it. That prompted an immediate step. After she completed each step, I said, "Good."

The completion phase started with a pause, which gave us both a chance to catch our breath. Then she continued by sliding her arm down to catch up with her feet. If she forgot to slide her hand down the banister, I gently moved it for her.

Stairs (up only)

In the second year of the dependent phase, June started having difficulty in climbing stairs. As we decreased drugs, her abilities improved. During the first two years of the final phase, she climbed the first two stairs with limited assistance, but needed extensive assistance for the remaining stairs. Even in the third year of the final phase, without prompting or assistance, she occasionally stepped up for the first stair or two. With prompting, she did it more frequently.

Getting on the bus

When June bumped against the back of a step, it prompted her to raise her foot. Because the bus had no riser, she walked under the step. I kept her back far enough so she could see the step. Then I prompted her with, "a big, high step." When she raised her foot enough, I helped her cover the extra distance.

After a hip replacement

After a hip replacement, one must relearn how to climb stairs.

▸ We went up before she became too tired. We approached the stairs with confidence and no hesitation. Whenever she raised a foot, I simultaneously took a step and lifted her arm. We developed a rhythm together, and our natural momentum helped her. Sometimes, she forgot to move her hand on the banister. So I moved her hand near a higher step as a prompt to step up.

▸ She reluctantly used the leg on the side of the hip replacement. For the last step, I took both of her hands in mine and turned her body to prompt her to lead with it. As her foot touched the top, I helped her to center her body so her weight was above her foot. That prevented her weight from pushing the knee off to the side. Then I stopped helping, and she used her own strength for the last step. That slowly strengthened her leg. After her leg became stronger, she could go up the stairs in about one minute.

Final Phase

As my wife weakened, the time to go up stairs gradually increased to fourteen minutes. To compensate, I developed three risky methods that allowed us to restore the time to ten minutes. As she continued to weaken, I realized I needed to find a better solution. I installed a stair lift. Since that solution was inevitable, I should have done it at the first sign of weakening. Although I do not recommend it, I am including the simplest of those three methods that one might consider using only until the stair lift is installed. This method required no weight-bearing use of my arms. Before using this method, one should carefully evaluate the risk. If one decides the risk is small, wear a transfer belt. Fasten it to the banister (and remove/refasten it every few steps).

▸ She stood next to and held the banister. I stood on her other side and positioned the shoulder of my touching arm in her armpit. A very slight lifting motion of my shoulder prompted her to step up.

Stair lift

We installed a stair lift in the third year of the final phase to get to and from the second floor. She got on the stair lift, scooted back, and held onto the arms without prompting or assistance. She got off without help. The lift eliminated safety concerns and allowed us to traverse the stairs in twenty-eight seconds.

▸ I brought her in from the side (so she did not have to back up) and positioned her where the lift would be. Then I brought the lift down to her, rotated its seat to the right position, and lowered its arms. The seat was too high for her to get seated properly, so I helped her scoot back. Then I lowered the foot-rest and placed her feet on it.

▸ As we moved, I kept one hand on the switch and my other arm across June. This gave her a secure feeling and acted as a restraint. For even greater safety, one can connect the safety belt on the stair lift. When we reached the top, I rotated the seat for her to get off.

▸ Coming down, one can position the lift so a person can get in easily.

Storage tip

Keeping a lift all the way up or down compresses and wears out the rubber bumper. When not in use, one will have more room by keeping it more out of the way.

WALKING

Dependent Phase

In the second year of this phase, June could still walk well. Only a year later, however, she could not walk alone safely. Drug side effects caused lower awareness and contributed to her first falls. When she tired, she also sometimes tried to sit with nothing behind her.

Away from home, we made good time if I held both of June's hands. She had more confidence when I did this, and she did not have a hand free to clutch anything. She acted more confident walking toward me, so I faced her and walked backwards. Sometimes, I walked beside her and reached across her front to hold her far hand. She could then hold my forearm with her other hand. Sometimes she attempted to get a hand (usually her left) out of mine. I thought she might have arthritis in that hand and treated it sparingly. After I released her hand once, however, she only wanted to scratch her nose. Whenever I felt resistance (what I called a stutter-step), we stopped. When she resumed, she took longer steps and we lost little time.

At home, she had great independence. However, I stayed close and watched her feet so she did not stub them. In bad weather, using the dry steps in the garage made falls less of a risk. Sometimes she attempted to go somewhere inappropriate. Rather than pull her back, I distracted her by getting between her and her objective.

If she stopped or pulled backwards, I let her pull me until I got close enough to give her a hug or kiss. She sometimes kissed me back, and we easily restarted.

Any drastic change in color or feel of the surface frightened her. She usually treated it as a step, so we stopped. She restarted when I told her it was flat and level and that she was "doing really well."

Final Phase

During the first two years of the final phase, June walked slowly with limited assistance. Her walking became shuffling, and neither foot left the ground completely. We avoided anything that might cause her to stumble. Since my daughter had a stone driveway, we parked on the grass when we visited. We could not avoid thresholds. She wrapped an arm around my shoulder, we took our time, and I talked her over them. We did not stop in doorways because she clutched both sides with viselike grips and reluctantly let go. Poor balance caused the day care staff to use two people to take her for walks. Holding her elbows, I rested her forearms on top of mine and encouraged her to hold tight. This enabled her to walk without additional help. Rocking from foot-to-foot or swiveling her hips from side to side could trigger starting. We repeated this slow procedure until we arrived at a nearby destination. Since she sometimes stepped on my feet and nearly caused falls, I walked with them out of harms way (both of my feet outside hers). It strained my arms when she leaned heavily on me, so we stopped until she stood upright. Those days, we paused every few feet to get her feet and body coordinated. She restarted easily with the prompt, "Ready?" If she ever needed to sit, I often zigzagged toward appropriate places.

During the last two years of the final phase, we had to pause after every few steps, and a turn required more maneuvering. I had to prompt her to move her feet constantly. We held each other's elbows for more support. Sometimes, her upper body moved but not her feet. She sometimes took a short right step, a normal left step, a short right step, and then rested before repeating the cycle. When I wanted a leg to move, I put a hand on her thigh or gently pushed from behind. As we went through narrow bathroom doors, we turned sideways to avoid crushed or bruised elbows and hands. An occasional bite on my shoulder took up to thirty days to heal. To avoid that, I made sure that either my shoulder fit under her chin or the side of her face fit snugly against my shoulder. In the evening, she was too tired to walk.

Turns

If we had lots of room, we made a slow curving turn as we walked. However, we often had little room. Under those circumstances late in the final phase, I imagined our turns resembling elephants dancing. With our arms around each other, we rocked from side to side, and her feet shifted with each rock. In her last year, her feet continued to go straight as we turned. Gentle pressure from my feet outside hers guided her feet through the turn.

Wheelchair

In the last year of the final phase, wheelchair transfers became the norm.

Getting into one from a car

▸ Lock the wheels so it cannot roll away. Position it facing the same direction as the car. The front should be at the midpoint of her seat so she does not have far to go.

▸ The footrests stuck out too far for her to back up between them. So she faced the seat and walked up to the wheelchair before turning to sit.

Moving from place to place

▸ Self-closing doors closed too quickly for our pace. Most residential doors have a closer shaft with a metal stopper that is easy to push up against the closer. Most commercial self-closing doors have a closer at the top of the door. A piece of metal is usually on the inside top of the door (near the hinge) with a small built-in lever. When raised to a horizontal position, it will hold the door open. For doors without a device to hold them open, one should slowly go through backwards.

▸ When passing anything solid that a person might cling to, slow to avoid breaking her arm. If a foot comes off a footrest, replace it immediately to avoid injuries.

▸ To prevent accidents, provide a restraint if one turns a family member's care over to others. They can more easily get a transfer belt on and off. Wrap it around the back and under the arms of the wheelchair to keep it from slipping up. One may also use a safety support vest. Wrap several loops of its straps around the back vertical poles. Put one strap snugly above and one snugly below the seat bar to assure they do not slip up.

Traversing a small step

Backing down is less physically demanding. Going up, however, one should go forward. Step on the projecting bar at the bottom rear of the wheelchair to raise the front enough to get past the step. That allows one's stronger feet to do the work instead of one's arms.

Traversing two steps

Tell your family member what is about to happen. Leaving the house, we went forward. Entering the house, we went backward. That way, one may safely tilt the wheelchair to balance its weight. The larger rear wheels roll over steps more easily. Do all movements slowly with constant reassurances.

One may also want to consider a ramp. A neighbor used two lightweight aluminum ramps (one for each wheel) that worked well for him. (See Products Chapter.)

Chapter 16
Other Tips

Bedroom

A family member needs a room to call her own, where she may rearrange things. The master bedroom may be the most familiar surrounding, and a place where she can be in charge.

▸ If someone eventually needs to move to another bedroom, it should be the caregiver. So a family member may have undisturbed rest, move a telephone (if any) too.

▸ Provide a safe environment (See that topic later in this chapter.)

▸ Opaque shades give the subdued lighting that encourages calmness.

▸ To help with incontinence accidents, place a long plastic runner along one side of the bed and another in the dressing area.

▸ After removing many things from the bedroom, little remains to touch, carry or hear. Put out soft clothes (socks, undershirts), photos, and perhaps a doll. Add a small radio tuned to a familiar station, and turn the volume low.

Bed

▸ To prevent mattresses from getting wet, cover them with a plastic garden cover before putting on a cloth mattress cover. Over that, overlap several highly absorbent washable underpads where her bottom rests.

▸ To provide warmth in the winter, use flannel sheets for the bed.

▸ If your family member gets in and out of bed frequently, remove covers during the day to reduce washing.

▸ Avoid using large blankets that one must take to a Laundromat for cleaning. Use several thinner blankets that one can wash at home.

When using a hospital bed

▶ If your family member spends much time in bed, use an egg crate pad and a massaging air mattress under the fitted sheet to prevent bedsores.

▶ To reduce bedding changes, use an incontinence draw sheet over the fitted sheet. In the later years, add a plain sheet, folded twice. Drape the longer ends off the sides to make it easier for care providers to move a person.

▶ To prevent arm bruises, tie a thick seat cushion to the side rails.

▶ If an illness is causing drainage from the mouth, roll your family member onto a side and wedge a pillow behind her back so she cannot roll back.

Bedtime

So your family member may sleep restfully, avoid strenuous exercise several hours before bedtime, serve a filling dinner, and do something relaxing afterwards. Unless one sees indications of fatigue, maintain a regular bedtime.

Preparation saves a last minute rush. Put an extra-absorbent insert in a fitted brief and lay out bedclothes. To compensate for tossed covers in the winter, use flannel clothes and include socks. If a severe weight loss has occurred, add lightweight glove liners. Lay out pills and prepare a toothbrush.

Putting to bed

▶ When a family member wears an identification bracelet, remove it to avoid accidents.

▶ If your family member sleeps on her back, keep covers loose by *tenting* them at toes and chest. To lessen the likelihood of uncovering, tuck the sheet under both arms.

▶ A person may scoot over the foot of the bed. She may then fall after becoming tangled in the covers. Angle her body across the bed slightly so she can scoot off the side and leave the sides of the covers loose.

▶ Slowly stroking the temple area with an electric massager (gentle setting) induces relaxation.

▶ We kept our home cool, especially at night. We preferred to use blankets to keep warm. To compensate for tossed covers in the winter, wait until she settles down before covering her. Whenever one awakes in the middle of the night, check to see that she has not uncovered herself. If your family member continually uncovers herself by morning and her skin is cool to your touch, raise the thermostat setting at night.

Behavioral changes

Many harmless changes will occur (e.g., setting the table with an extra place setting, or closing all of the drapes during the day). It helps to understand the reasons for common actions so one may have the proper level of empathy for a family member.

▸ They ask repetitive questions not because they didn't pay attention to an answer, but because they have probably forgotten that they asked the question.

▸ When they say, "I want to go home," their mind is probably on an earlier home in their life.

▸ With money in their wallets, "I don't have any money" probably means, "I feel that I have lost my independence."

▸ Other changes may show underlying problems, which one must uncover. Agitation (e.g., rapidly patting a table) may show frustration with the inability to deal with or explain a problem. When the caregiver fails to respond to someone's discomfort, even more behavioral changes, such as clutching, may result.

Agitation

If agitation or other indications do not stem from obvious stimuli, a caregiver needs to consider whether a family member:

▸ Needs companionship.

▸ Is thirsty, hungry, or in pain.

▸ Has a need to use the toilet or requires a change of clothes.

▸ Is too hot or too cold.

▸ Hears a loud noise or is upset by visitors.

▸ Is in uncomfortable or unfamiliar surroundings.

▸ Is in the early cycle of new pills and the dosage level may be incorrect.

Start with the most frequent cause of problems and work your way down the list.

▸ Give your family member attention, affection, and a drink.

▸ Tend to any bathroom needs. Change clothing if necessary.

▸ Adjust the room temperature.

▸ Eliminate any noise and distractions.

▸ Modify surroundings.

▸ Take your family member for a walk or listen to music.

▸ If one cannot determine the cause of the problem, evaluate whether the agitation justifies calling a doctor.

Clutching

A family member who enjoys a warming touch may also like to hold hands or have other physical contact with another person. As dementia sets in, judgment may wane and inappropriate touching of others may occur, including strangers. A *touching* person may become a *tightly clutching* person. It may not endear them to others. Some care providers may report this as aggressive behavior and suggest increased medication. Ignore that suggestion temporarily in favor of these ideas.

> ‣ Teach persons she offends to say, "Excuse me," quickly followed by, "Thank you," as they slowly remove a hand.
> ‣ As a way to help maintain balance when standing, encourage clutching something solid. Holding hands may also provide both affection and reassurance.

Hiding items

Many items may disappear and wind up in inappropriate places, especially during the early years. Sorting through the trash and the recycle bins will not be your favorite pastime.

> ‣ To avoid that onerous task, leave a bin in an obvious place for your family member to put things in and keep a hidden bin for the real trash.
> ‣ Also, check the garbage disposal before using it

Scooting

Ill persons may scoot off whatever they are lying or sitting on, become wedged between heavy furniture, and a serious injury may occur.

> ‣ At the first sign of scooting, get them up from their current position. They are probably tired of that position, so try going for a walk.
> ‣ If scooting recurs, consider the same causes as for agitation.

Calendars

Each spouse usually keeps their own calendar for appointments, reminders, etc. As I merged both of our calendars into one, it left no room for illness-related activities. We needed two additional month-at-a-glance calendars. I kept them in the handiest place so I could record data as I walked by. To make data easier to find, each calendar can have a different use.

> ‣ Use one for scheduled respite, day care transportation, and tax-deductible expenses. One may record day care attendance by

highlighting the date with a marker. Note exceptions to hours and holiday dates. Use as a reminder of day care events, requests, and due dates (payments, fitted brief orders, and bus trip cancellations).

▸ Use the other for daily care. One may record changes in medicine, dosages, and incontinence data. This will be useful in reporting to doctors and evaluating your progress in maintaining continence.

Communications, oral (Also see Vocabulary, Appendix K)

Throughout the companionship phase, June asked the same question repeatedly. Write the question and an answer on a piece of paper. She might then carry this paper with her and repeatedly read the answer.

In the later phases, June usually only talked to me—perhaps in response to my frequent comments. Her speech decreased dramatically, however, when she became ill or took medicine to reduce the effects of the dementia. To gauge the progress of her illness, I frequently asked, "What is your name?" At the beginning of the dependent phase, she could give her full-married name. By the middle of that phase, she gave her full birth name or first name only. By the end of that phase, she did not respond. When feeding ice cream (her favorite food), I asked if it were good. Through that phase, she usually gave an enthusiastic, "Yes." Early in the final phase, she still gave a pleased sound.

Increasing communication

Communications can be similar to two ships passing in the night.

▸ Create the proper environment—quiet, no one else around, gently holding a hand.

▸ Gain and keep attention by using her name, sitting close, and looking directly at her.

▸ Use the same words as one would with any other adult.

▸ Talk about your children. Reminisce about the good times, treasured moments, and the wonderful qualities of your family member.

▸ Have empathy and express sympathy if one suspects the slightest discomfort.

▸ By keeping one's tone of voice mild, the demeanor of a family member remains calm. Dementia does not infer deafness. My wife's reactions showed that she understood everything said in normal tones. (When a nurse spoke loudly to her in the final phase, June told her to shut up.)

Notes

▶ A person enjoys terms of endearment. Speak slowly and pause after each sentence.

▶ Use short words and sentences. Limit conversations to a few sentences.

▶ Assume that she understands all or part of what one says.

▶ Give a cheerful good morning on awakening. Sit together before arising. I usually said, "Hi, it's Frank," and talked for a few minutes.

▶ Repeat oneself. At bedtime, I said goodnights in a dozen different ways until she recognized a familiar phrase. (She last responded near the end of the dependent phase.)

▶ Respond to what she says, but also to what she feels or means.

▶ After a pleased sound, try, "I'm glad you're happy."

▶ Don't disagree. Try, "Yes, and let's . . . first."

▶ Respond positively to everything (even if indecipherable). If she said, "Thank you," even when I had done nothing, I still said, "You're welcome." When she said, "I want to go home," I said, "OK, may I go with you?" Then she smiled and said, "Yes." If she said, "You're stupid," I said, "You're right." Then we had a good laugh together.

"Find the good and praise it."—Alex Haley

In spite of limited abilities, family members try very hard. Encourage them during and praise them after a situation. These typical compliments often brought smiles or other responses:

▶ "You are so good."

▶ "I am very proud of you."

▶ After climbing the stairs—"Good job."

▶ If she raised her arms to help undress—"You are very helpful."

▶ When she lifted a foot to put into her pants—"That was very good."

▶ After getting dressed—"You look very good."

▶ When I complimented her, I often patted her on the shoulder, and she said, "Thank you." If I just patted her on the shoulder, she sometimes still said, "Thank you."

Explain what and why

Before we did anything, I used verbal preparation. Thus, I didn't surprise her, and she cooperated more easily.

▶ Upon arising—"We're going to take your night gown off to put on some dry clothes." For other tasks—"Let's get ready to . . ." On the other hand, I avoided telling her we were getting ready for something she might not enjoy. Instead, I said, "Let's get ready for some juice" (which she loved after anything).

▸ While dressing early in the illness, I walked her through each step, sometimes repeating the instructions.

▸ Whenever I left her side, I told her my destination and purpose. "I am going to the kitchen to warm your ice cream. I'll be right back."

Stimulating/preventing action

▸ Save the action request for last—"Here is your pill. Open your mouth." She usually responded positively within my first three requests.

▸ If possible, limit imperatives to one word.

▸ June had a strong grip. Occasionally, she held something that I wanted her to release. Pretending that she was handing it to me, I said, "Thank you" while reaching for it. Then she released it.

▸ When I told her what not to do, she usually forgot the negative. Stating things positively got better results. If a person starts to sit with nothing behind her, say *stand up*, rather than *don't sit*.

Double meanings

I learned the hard way not to use certain words or expressions that had double meanings.

▸ After a satisfactory result, I sometimes said, "There we go." She then became impatient to go somewhere. Ditto for "Let go."

▸ While changing her fitted briefs, she sometimes became impatient, and I said, "Hold on." Once, she clutched my ears and held tightly until I could eventually free one of my hands.

Final phase

As awareness declines, oral communications will become more one-sided. June seldom spoke except in response to me or to seeing a child or animal on television. One exception occurred in the second year of the final phase. She spoke three long and intelligent sentences that swept away the vestiges of her illness. It left me in awe for several days.

▸ Ask a person questions that only require a one-word response.

▸ If no response, repeat the question more slowly.

▸ By the second year of the final phase, her responses might come several minutes after a question. Give lots of time for a response and wait until she finishes.

▸ Stand close and listen carefully because responses may be barely audible.

‣ If I didn't understand something she said, I repeated it, sometimes with a slight rephrasing to make sure that I understood.

‣ I learned to interpret the tiniest part of a phrase. "Pl . . . " asked me to do or not do something.

‣ Even if she said something unintelligible, I responded with, "Yes," and tried to prolong the conversation.

‣ In the last few years, June seldom answered, nodded, or turned her head toward me. Nevertheless, I spoke to her the same way, hoping she understood some of what I said.

‣ Caregivers in this stage should see the inspiring Spanish movie *Talk to Her*. Director Pedro Almodovar got an Oscar nomination for his story of two men and the two comatose women they loved.

Advice to others who provide care

‣ Introduce yourself at each meeting. (Do not assume a person remembers your last visit.)

‣ Do not speak about a patient to someone else in his or her presence. Instead, address her directly. If she cannot respond, then the caregiver will help.

‣ Very young care providers should experiment to see whether an older patient prefers that one call her by her first or last name.

Communications, body language

June appreciated touching, and I assumed that she had a high awareness level.

‣ When I walked by, I gave her a hug or a kiss (better than a dozen possibly misunderstood statements). Sometimes she responded with a smile.

‣ While giving hugs to each other, I patted her back with my right hand. Sometimes, she responded by patting my back.

‣ Any time she glanced at me, I smiled at her. Occasionally, she smiled back. Other times, she just looked grateful.

She often telegraphed what she wanted or planned to do. I only needed to concentrate on the appropriate body part.

‣ Her feet told me to anticipate movement on the stairs. Uncrossing her legs while seated often showed preparation to get up.

‣ If she put her hand into her mouth, it usually showed hunger. Opening her mouth during a meal meant she was ready for more.

‣ Holding something out in front of her showed that she was about to drop it on the floor.

▶ Clasping her arms across her chest showed she was not interested in continuing her current activity.

▶ In the final phase, June's prevalent form of *negative* non-oral communication was agitation. Once, my daughter and her family came to visit. When a grandson fell off his bicycle and bloodied his face, she spilled her juice on the floor for the only time that year.

▶ As late as her final year, she acknowledged compliments, kisses, terms of endearment, and greetings with a smile. Occasionally, she nodded her head in agreement and sometimes widened her eyes with pleasure. Once, she pressed her lips against my cheek when I asked for a kiss.

▶ Sometimes she burst into laughter, which made me smile. My smile encouraged her to laugh more and soon, I began laughing too. After we finished laughing, she smiled, and we both felt better. It was an activity that we could share.

Constipation, easing

June became uncomfortable if she did not maintain a regular schedule. At home, she had no trouble. It usually became a problem after a respite stay at a nursing facility. It took up to four days to get her back to normal.

▶ The first morning after her return, I gave her two glasses of water and 3-5 prunes. (Prunes are high in antioxidants that reduce the activity of cell-damaging free radicals.) Then I added a tablespoon of olive oil to each meal and increased the number of times she spent on the toilet.

▶ In addition, I asked the day-care center staff to increase the liquids they gave.

▶ If those things did not work, I added a small can of prune juice daily.

▶ Meanwhile, it eased her discomfort and made a bowel movement easier if she slept on her side rather than her back.

Driving, stopping

Driving represents independence. Family members will usually lose the spatial skills required for driving years before they lose their awareness skills. Do not count on your ability to check driving habits by a test ride. Since problems may be intermittent, it could be one of the few safe trips. Removing driving privileges is one of the most heart-wrenching decisions a caregiver must make. Leading up to this decision, however, many warning signs occur:

- Not being alert about where walking
- Concern from doctors about spatial relationships
- Not being able to find where she parked the car
- Failure to drive defensively or involvement in a minor accident
- Lack of confidence when driving (e.g., reluctance to drive out of the local area, or abandoning the car in bad weather)

What to try first

- Review the reasons for your family member driving.
- Assume chores they may not enjoy, such as banking.
- Do as many things as possible together—the library, sightseeing, shopping for clothes and groceries. Attend the same religious services. Get your haircuts simultaneously.
- If being alone at a destination is more appropriate for your family member (e.g., a social engagement), volunteer to drive to and from the event. (Your family member will probably enjoy having your company.)
- Talk about self-restricting driving in certain situations (e.g., no driving at night or in bad weather). One should also broach the subject of not driving at all.

Stopping driving

The above steps should dramatically reduce family members' driving, and they may even have lost some desire to drive. As the warning signs increase (e.g., new dents or scrapes) or one gets a call from a neighbor about observed dangerous behavior, family members should stop driving.

- Discuss the reasons for stopping with your family member. Blame the disease, not them.
- Consider having your doctor write a *stop-driving* prescription.
- Let her keep her license—and her dignity. It is a good form of identification.
- Hiding the keys in one's home is not a good idea. (A family member can be very resourceful at times.) Instead, keep the keys on your person.
- When seeing their car becomes too painful for your family member, sell it.

Other sources

A booklet, *We Need to Talk*, is available from The Hartford [insurance company], 200 Executive Blvd., Southington, CT 06489. AARP worked with them to produce it. The Winter 2004 edition of

USAA [insurance company] Magazine also listed a five-step plan from the American Medical Association.

▸ Tell your family member about one's concerns.
▸ Help create a transportation plan.
▸ Help reduce driving.
▸ Encourage a visit to the doctor.
▸ Suggest a driving test.

Emergency information

Keep emergency medical data for yourself in your wallet. Your family member should also carry emergency information. Post a copy on your refrigerator. Include utility repair numbers for others who provide care. (See Appendix F)

Exercise

Through the second year of the dependent phase, June exercised without my help. She spent most of her time at day care pacing up and down the halls. The day-care center also did range-of-motion (stretching) exercises.

▸ To create an area where a person can safely walk by herself at home, close off several rooms and move furniture to enlarge paths. While she walks, one should sit nearby.
▸ Exercise may be done together, which makes it more enjoyable. Instead of calling it exercise, say, "Would you like to go for a walk?" (We toured a seven-room path through the house several times a day. Each lap included going into and out of a sunken living room.) To increase normal exercise, one should walk to all destinations by the longest route.
▸ Climbing stairs strengthens one's legs. (After returning from nursing facilities, it took up to twice the length of her stay there to regain her strength.)

After a hip replacement

For four months, she spent part of the time in a wheelchair. After she returned from day care, we walked around the house at least three times. After she stopped using the wheelchair, we gradually increased the number of times that she climbed stairs. She had to work hard at first, and she was almost out of breath when we reached the top. By the time that we did fifty stairs daily, however, she was in much better shape. In five months, she could climb all fourteen stairs, alternating feet, without stopping. It took another three months before she did it regularly. Our walks lasted up to twenty-five minutes.

Stretching

▸ Stretch at times when your family member is already in the correct position. When she is lying down, keep each leg straight and raise it as high as it will go. When sitting (while drying or putting on shoes), bend her knee and raise her leg as high as it will go. With the leg straight out, rest a foot on your thigh (another stretch) before raising the second leg.

▸ Stretch slowly to prevent injuries and hold each position for a slow count of thirty.

▸ Try three repetitions of each stretch three times a day.

▸ To prevent a leg from turning in, loosen the abductor muscles of the inner thigh by stretching and holding both legs apart.

▸ To learn more about stretching, one may want to read the book, *Stretching*, by Bob and Jean Anderson.

LESSONS LEARNED

Recovery time increases as one gets older. Except normal exercise (walking), it may take several days to recover. It may take a week to adjust to a higher level of exercise. For strenuous exercises, do them more slowly.

Falls, preventing

While taking drugs, a family member becomes a strong candidate for falls. After June's broken hip, the social worker at the rehabilitation center did a *Falling Risk Assessment* using a scale of 0-34. They considered any number greater than nine a risk, and June scored twenty-one.

▸ Fall proof one's home. (See Safety in this chapter.)

▸ A family member should wear shoes that fit well with flat, non-slip soles.

▸ If family members' medicine makes them drowsy, never leave them alone during waking hours. If one needs a few minutes alone, put her in a geriatric chair in front of the television.

▸ Since an imbalance and a fall can happen in an instant, hold on to each other when standing or walking.

▸ Do not let her hold hands with herself. It fools her into thinking she is safe.

▸ If family members move around a lot after major surgery, take precautions at bedtime until they heal. Use a safety support vest tied to the bed frame. After one has gained enough confidence that they will not hurt themselves (four months in my case), one may delay tying it until they fall asleep. Once they are not as active (two more months in my case), one may have enough confidence to stop using it.

Feet and nail care

Some of June's toenails became misshapen and extremely thick. She also lost the nail on her right great toe at a nursing facility. A podiatrist said he feared getting hurt by her sudden movements and could not guarantee removing two corns. At a nursing facility, she developed a rash (athletes' foot) between her toes. In the final phase, she got a foot ulcer on the back of a heel.

LESSONS LEARNED

- ▸ For all lengthy procedures (nail care), choose a day when one will not have to rush (e.g., a weekend). Pick the calmest time of the day (e.g., after morning juice or dinner).
- ▸ Have a comfortable place for your family member to sit. An overstuffed chair or couch works when caring for the feet. A geriatric chair works better for cutting fingernails.
- ▸ Have a comfortable place for yourself to sit on both sides of your family member. Something moveable (a hassock) works well. That allows one to sit close to the side on which one is working.
- ▸ Cut all nails short regularly. That will prevent self-scratches from fingernails and toenails from being torn off while donning pants.
- ▸ Rest the entire arm or leg comfortably. A family member moves an arm more slowly when it is resting on the tray of the geriatric chair. Propping a leg straight out on one's knee helps reduce leg movement.
- ▸ For a corn, soak the foot in warm water until the corn softens. Then scoop it out. If one has a pedicure clipper with a scoop on the end, one can easily do this.
- ▸ Work on a toe rash after a bath. Pat dry and then use a blow dryer. Rub baby powder across and down between the toes. Within two weeks, the rash should heal.
- ▸ A foot ulcer requires frequent podiatrist visits. At home, soak the heel twice a day with a warm Domeboro solution. Buy a heel boot (See Products Chapter), for your family member to wear while in bed.
- ▸ Have patience. It may take months for some areas to heal. For nails, it may take years for them to return to normal.

Hair appointments

Through the companionship phase, June cooperated in getting her hair done, and I had my hair cut simultaneously. When she finished early, a stylist (whose father had Alzheimer's disease) held hands with her until I finished. During the dependent phase, June had trouble holding still and staying seated. Since a trip to the salon lifted her spirits, we had to make it work.

Getting ready
▸ To reduce the time with the stylist, I washed June's hair beforehand.
▸ During a period of increased agitation in the dependent phase, I gave June a little extra antianxiety medication beforehand. Once, I forgot, and she became very fidgety. When I apologized, the stylist said, "Oh, she was much worse a couple of years ago."
▸ Our shop did not make appointments. To cut down on June's agitation, I called the day before to see if her stylist would be in. If so, I canceled June's day care bus pickup. Early the next day, I called the stylist, and she agreed to sign June in and told me when we should arrive.

Getting hair done
▸ So I could calm June while the stylist cut her hair, I got my hair cut at a different time.
▸ The stylist cut her hair short to make it easier to provide care.
▸ Under hospice care, I became her stylist. Besides the hair cutting equipment, I used pinking shears to avoid a *cut* look.

Hands, washing/wiping
▸ June did little to get her hands dirty, so we only washed before meals, at bedtime, and after her return from day-care.
▸ To mimic her own habits, we washed both her hands simultaneously at a bathroom sink. After she had trouble bending over, we washed at the higher kitchen sink. She stood sideways, and we did them singly. Facing each another, I soaped one of my hands and washed her opposite hand. Then we reversed sides.
▸ After meals, I used a wet washcloth to wipe her hands and mouth. I learned to wipe food from her hands quickly. (Once, she shoved food deep into her nose.)

▶ After wiping her face, I untied her bib and gradually rolled it down after unclasping and wiping the messier hand. If I took too long to wipe her second hand, she re-clasped her hands, so I held one until I finished with the other.

▶ She reacted more positively if I told her what I planned and if I picked up her hands slowly and wiped them gently. I usually said, "Excuse me," just before I did that.

Laundry

June did the laundry alone through the independent phase. During the companionship phase, I only helped with the proper washer/dryer settings, which I did inconspicuously. So with little supervision, she could manage. This low risk activity gave her much pleasure. It did not matter if clothes later wound up in the wrong drawers.

Later phases

▶ The most convenient time to wash was after changing clothes in the morning. If incontinence affected clothes, I used the hot setting, did some separately, and used a second rinse cycle.

▶ When I did the sheets, I threw the plastic underpad in for the first minutes of the wash cycle. Then I rinsed it manually and hung it out to dry.

Liquids

Early Phases

June helped herself to liquids. We also had a relaxing glass of wine at dinnertime. Drugs made her too sleepy after the companionship phase, however, and I stopped giving wine to her.

Early Dependent Phase

June could drink without assistance, but could not show her thirst. We both drank a large glass (14 oz.) of water upon arising. She also had a small glass at meals and after brushing her teeth. Giving water while toileting sometimes acted as a trigger and it didn't matter if it spilled. Also, I gave her water whenever I drank and anytime she awoke and fussed. She drank a small glass before leaving for day-care and after her return. At lunch, I served a small glass of milk and a large bowl of soup.

She drank more when seated. The geriatric chair (with the tray up) kept her seated until she finished and gave her a place to rest her glass.

Late Dependent Phase

June could drink alone, but spilt much of the liquid. Usually, she took a long sip immediately after I handed her a drink. Most spills followed a long pause. So I took the drink out of her hand and gave her short rests between sips. If she set the drink down on the tray, I removed it temporarily so she did not accidentally knock it over. Filling her glass ½ to ¾ full gave her enough so she did not have to tilt the glass far, but not enough to spill easily.

To decrease spillage, I switched to cups with lids and tiny holes. I kept one in her bedroom. That helped with middle-of-the-night drinks in bed. Trying to get her to use the cup handles ended in spillage. Instead, I curled her hand around the cup close to the bottom. Then I guided the cup to her mouth until she tilted it, which helped her remember how. When she had trouble tilting her head far enough back to drink, I gently tilted the cup. To remind her how to raise her arm from the tray to lift the cup, I prompted her by gently lifting her elbow.

After a while, she could no longer find the tiny hole in the lid of the cup. So I switched to seven-ounce juice glasses because she could wrap her whole hand around them and hold them securely. Lightweight plastic glasses did not tire her, and did not break when dropped on the tiled bathroom floor. To make sure she knew that she held a glass, I watched until she took the first sip. If not, I tilted the glass. If she released the glass, I held it but wrapped her hand around mine to get her used to the motion.

Final Phase

Since she had trouble tilting her head back, she could drink water more easily with a full glass. Otherwise, a glass with a wide brim works well because one can tilt it without hitting one's nose.

If June became drowsy, choking became a concern. Using flexible straws caused her to participate and kept her awake. Wetting her lips with the liquid motivated her to start sucking, especially something tasty. If that did not work, I slowly withdrew the straw. Trying to retain the straw caused her to resume sucking.

LESSON LEARNED

▸ Lots of liquids helped to prevent urinary tract infections.

Quiet time

Parents with small children understand the need for quiet time. Long caregiving days prompted my memory. In the dependent phase, I scheduled one-half hour (later one hour) after breakfast. June paced in her room with the door closed, but usually laid down. On the weekends, I added a second period in the late afternoon, but got her up at the first sign of movement. For four and one-half months after her hip replacement, the safety support vest kept her from injuring herself.

In the final phase, we had quiet times of about three hours, split between morning and afternoon. She listened to soft rock or classical music on the radio, with the volume low.

Recreation

Independent Phase

Within the limits of my job, we started doing many things that we had postponed. We had at least one travel adventure each year. On my longer business trips, I took June along. We bought a bicycle for June, and we explored the Washington & Old Dominion bike trail from Washington, D.C. to Purcellville, Virginia. For eleven years, we had talked about visiting the White House at Christmas. In spite of the cold, we enjoyed the camaraderie of the others waiting in a long line, and the beautiful candle lit rooms.

We also made June's in-house stays at NIH as pleasant as possible. While I ate my dinner in the cafeteria, she had an extra dessert. Then we walked in the beautiful walled-in garden. After each stay, I planned a short vacation at nearby country inns in Annapolis, Baltimore, Cape May, Charles Town, or Gettysburg.

Companionship Phase

I looked upon these years as our last chance to do many things. My sister accompanied us on a month-long trip to the northwestern United States and Canada to visit cousins. When friends moved to Italy, we braved a month-long trip there. On a leisurely drive via the Blue Ridge Parkway, we stayed at all three inns. As a transition from June's cooking to mine, we ate out three times a week at local restaurants. On June's birthday, we ate at favorite restaurants—L'Auberge Chez Francois or the Inn at Little Washington. When Dick Francis signed his books in Middleburg, we also had lunch there.

Later Phases

June could no longer participate in most of the activities at the day-care center. In a search for something that might please her, I tested her reaction to all of our cable channels. Nature programs and music prompted the most positive responses. Because country music played continuously, we watched it more often. She relaxed more if we kept the volume turned low. She sometimes smiled, clapped, tapped her feet, and wiggled her toes. Once, she said, "That was good." It pleased me when we could enjoy something together.

LESSON LEARNED
▸ Don't postpone fun.

Routines

June found it difficult to cope with change. Once, I offered her pills while she sat on her bed, and she refused to take them. After I led her to her sink where I usually gave them, she accepted them readily. After her hip replacement, she became upset when she could not have breakfast where she normally ate—in her geriatric chair. She felt more comfortable when I maintained routines. When I did them in the same way on the same schedule, she readily helped. Even as late as the beginning of the final phase, she anticipated the next step in a sequence and did it before I asked.

My own routines made it easier to handle things when something unusual happened. When I flew in the Air Force, we practiced our routines endlessly. In times of emergency, our minds went on *autopilot* to accomplish them. After long respites, I sometimes forgot steps in a sequence. In stressful caregiving situations, only the *autopilot* of the routine assured things got done. For tasks that did not have a daily routine, I used reminders. I left lights on to remind me to do something in a particular room, such as handle laundry. If I started a new routine, I put a reminder in an unusual place. After June's hip replacement, I kept forgetting her safety vest. So I put it on the floor in a path I had to take. If we needed my car to do something, I put a note on my car seat. Building slack for the unexpected into each routine reduced stress.

In a normal week, June needed sixty-six hours of care. We averaged more because of holidays and snow days. Non-caregiving chores added about twenty hours weekly. The longest period without respite occurred during the big blizzards of 1996. She stayed home for more than nine days. Routines allowed me to be more efficient because I did not have to stop and think as often.

Mornings

The morning routine started when we arose and lasted until June left for day-care. In the dependent phase, it took about two hours.

That gradually increased to four and one-half to five hours by the final phase.

- ► Early mornings (ninety minutes) included eating and exercising.
- ► Quiet time in her room (ninety minutes). First-aid chores sometimes took the entire period.
- ► Late mornings (ninety minutes) included bathing, dressing, drinking juice, and exercising.
- ► The bus took her to day care. (If I had to drive her, it took a total of thirty-minutes.)

Evenings

The evening routine started when June came home from day-care and lasted until she went to bed. It normally took three hours, but could take up to four and one-half hours. During the dependent phase, it included exercise, juice, and dinner (seventy minutes), television (half hour), preparing for bed and first aid (ninety minutes).

In the final phase, June usually fell asleep early, so we ate when she got off the bus. Dinner could take much longer. (On a slow day, it took her up to forty seconds to chew and swallow a mouthful.) If she were sleepier than usual, she only had juice and a little food. I compensated on the weekends by increasing the quantity of lunch. By the middle of this phase, she became too tired to stay up after dinner.

Weekends

We expanded all activities to fill the extra five afternoon hours. I saved her shampoo and a full bath until then. Because we did not hurry, it was a pleasant experience for both of us. Both days, I increased quiet time and added more exercise. I added variety to our liquids with freshly brewed tea mixes from homegrown herbs. After lunch, I brushed her teeth an extra time. After quiet time, we expanded our juice/TV time. To prolong these mellow times, I seated her in an easy chair next to a large picture window that had a good view of the bird feeders in our yard.

Holidays

The day care center had ten holidays yearly, which sometimes resulted in five three-day weekends and two four-day weekends. A plan for dealing with these long weekends made them more relaxing. Our family invited us out for special holidays. I used more pre-cooked meals and sometimes ordered pizza. To make one day fly by, we enjoyed driving in the country, buying fruit at farm stands, or walking in the park. Various other errands got us out of the house and helped take away a trapped feeling.

My routines

Each morning, I prepared breakfast to give the house a chance to warm before I got June up. Weekdays, the only *quiet time* followed breakfast. When the day care bus pulled away with June on it, I felt relieved. I finished the hectic chores early. So I would not have to rush after she came home, I did as much as possible beforehand. To give me time to wind down, I saved an hour to shower, and relax while reading short stories and drinking hot herbal tea.

During her quiet times on weekends, I usually relaxed and rested too. For long weekends, I sometimes saved a one-time project, for which I did the preparation during the week. Then I looked forward to completing the job.

While she watched television after dinner, I sat on the couch near her doing things that I could easily interrupt and restart. After I put June to bed, I looked forward to relaxing and watching a movie from my tape collection.

Safety

▸ Prepare for an emergency. Keep emergency numbers by a telephone on each floor. Install one telephone next to your bed. Keep working flashlights where one is most likely to be if electricity goes out, especially next to one's bed. Give spare house keys to family and neighbors. Make sure that your home address is clearly visible from both directions of the street at night. (Large black numbers on both sides of a white mailbox should work nicely.)

▸ Decrease the chance of a fall. Drastically reduce the items of furniture and accumulated *stuff*. Move the rest far enough apart so your family member may easily navigate through the home. Get rid of slippery throw rugs. Clear floors of clutter—including indoor plants. Store the remainder in closets or drawers. Keep rooms well lit.

▸ To prevent a family member from pulling or knocking them down, remove pictures from a wall that she passes (e.g., stairway).

▸ Family members may lock themselves in a room without a second exit (e.g., bedroom or bathroom). Keep a tool handy that will allow *picking* inside door locks. Better still (and less stressful), remove the inside lock.

▸ Install childproof locks on appropriate cabinets and high catches on the doors to the furnace and tool rooms. For offices, use locking cabinets and boxes. To avoid your family member eating or hiding pills, store them in a safe place. Put breakables in an inaccessible place. If one has guns in the house, store the ammunition elsewhere.

Bath

▸ Replace worn non-slip surfaces in the tubs or add a non-slip rubber mat (with suction cups on the bottom).
▸ Install grab bars in appropriate places.
▸ Switch to liquid soap. (June ate bar soap.)
▸ Clear clutter from the toilet tank top and sink vanities.

Bedroom/dressing area

▸ Rugs should be wall-to-wall or non-slip.
▸ In the closets, store only clothes and items that cannot harm a person.
▸ Remove breakable lamps and pictures protected with glass. Isolate or remove furniture with sharp corners that might cause an injury during a fall (e.g., a nightstand).
▸ Get rid of anything drinkable (including household products and perfume) and anything else that a family member might accidentally swallow. Remove anything chewable from both the top and inside vanities—including removable plastic towel racks. The space that one has created will provide storage for dental and incontinence supplies.

Electrical

▸ Cover the open electrical outlets with plastic inserts. For areas with running water, install Ground Fault Interrupted wall outlets with a reset button.
▸ Run electrical cords behind furniture or fasten them to the walls. Use cord shorteners to get rid of excess cord.
▸ If one has convenient circuit breakers, trip the stove breaker between meals. (If one has a gas stove, remove the burner knobs.)
▸ Turn the hot water heater temperature down to 120 degrees. (Since that setting will not sanitize dishes, use the high temperature setting on your dishwasher.)
▸ Unplug the microwave, toaster, and coffee maker. (When others provide care, consider also unplugging the kitchen disposal.) Unplug or store a blow dryer.

▶ For light fixtures that a person might touch, use burn-cool bulbs.

▶ Keep a night light in bathrooms, stairways, and the bedroom of your family member. (If one is forgetful, buy timers for them.)

▶ In each bedroom and at the top and bottom of stairs, install either glow-in-the-dark light switches or put glow-in-the-dark stickers on the switch plate.

Fire

▶ Move the bedroom of your family member to the first floor near one, and preferably two, outside exits.

▶ Check with your fire department to see if they will do a free safety check. (Ask if any other local services offer free safety checks.)

▶ To give maximum lead-time for a slow-moving person, install a smoke detector on every floor, including the basement.

▶ Keep fire extinguishers in handy places on each floor—near the stove, furnace, storage areas, bathrooms, and automobiles.

▶ Have your chimneys cleaned regularly.

Kitchen

▶ Store any food out of reach. (One day, I found June chewing the hard banana skin end with no trace of the rest of the skin.) Only have items on the kitchen counter that have high usage. Do not store items in the oven. (Having fewer things around will allow one to more closely monitor the rest.)

▶ Although I stored it on a high shelf, I still got rid of our liquor supply.

▶ Put any knives and scissors in a safe place.

▶ Since getting distracted with a caregiving task is easy, use a reminder when cooking something on the stove. (I pinned a bright red potholder on my belt loop.) Keep all pot handles turned in.

Poison

▶ Dispose of old prescriptions.

▶ Store other toxic items (cleaning supplies, pesticides, medicine chest items, etc.) in an inaccessible place. (I used a very high shelf in the laundry room.)

▶ Check for toxic houseplants.

▶ Buy those products that have safety packaging, such as childproof caps.

▶ Although the phone book has the Poison Control Center telephone number on the first page, also put it on each phone.

Other source

Call the U.S. Consumer Product Safety Commission (Washington, D.C. 20207) at 800-638-2772 (hearing-impaired 800-638-8270). Ask for their free safety booklets (electrical audit, fire, home wiring, and poison).

Skills, maintaining

For ill persons to maintain their dignity, they need to function at the boundaries of their abilities. When my efforts flagged once, the sight of a dementia patient at a nursing facility trying to eat soup with her fingers inspired me. To gain a better appreciation of the effort required for a simple task, I analyzed the number of mental and physical steps it took to cut and eat a piece of meat. It required fifteen steps in the proper sequence—a hard task for someone with dementia.

▶ My communications reflected our sharing tasks. In the companionship phase, I said, "May I help?" Later, "Let me help." Finally, "Would you like to help?" My talking frequently prompted her to maintain her own speech skills.

▶ By working together, June maintained skills in all areas—even in the final phase. (See earlier chapters, the Communications topic in this chapter, Assumption #4 in Chapter 17, Vocabulary in Appendix K, and Independent skills in Appendix L.)

LESSONS LEARNED

▶ Be patient. Waiting to help may give your family member the extra time needed to do the task.

▶ Build extra time into schedules. That will help resist the temptation to help too soon.

▶ Prompts work (I have listed many in this chapter and the previous five chapters).

▶ A family member may succeed in regaining skills, especially after doctors have decreased or eliminated a medicine.

Travel

▶ Plan enough slack time into each day so it is leisurely.

▶ Prepare for emergencies. Carry emergency information cards that include medical conditions and references to each other. Carry a cell phone.

▸ Wear matching caps, tops, and jackets so that others may easily identify you as together.

▸ Use unisex bathrooms together. (Most service stations and bathrooms for the disabled in airports have them.) If one must use separate bathrooms, find an attendant of the same sex who will watch over your family member until reunited.

Driving

▸ Join AAA or a similar organization.

▸ Plan no more than six hours of driving (about three hundred miles).

▸ Do not take long trips in winter or drive at night. Carry water. Start early enough in the morning to get to your lodging in time to relax before dinner.

Flying

▸ Use nonstop flights.

▸ Keep in close physical contact in the terminals by holding hands.

Lodgings

▸ Avoid staying in rooms that one must enter from outside the building. The corridor to your room should lead to an attended front desk.

▸ To alert one to wandering in the middle of the night, use all locks on your door. Then wedge a chair under the doorknob or place a heavy object in front of the door.

▸ If a room has two beds, sleep nearest the door.

▸ Bring your own night-light for the bathroom.

Wandering, preventing

At home

▸ Cut down on urges to wander by creating an atmosphere of calm, getting much exercise, and having some form of recreation.

▸ Install window locks and keyed dead bolts on the doors (see Products Chapter). Keep the keys handy (but out of sight) during the day. Put the keys back into the doors at night. To guard against accidentally locking oneself out (with your family member inside), keep your keys on your person—even to get the mail. As your family member's awareness declines, keys may be kept in the doors.

▸ A tall lightweight chair sideways in a bedroom doorway will normally prevent exiting. If not, one can easily exchange the inside locking door handle/knob for the outside one that does not lock. Locking the bedroom door after bedtime will prevent exiting (and perhaps an accidental fall down the stairs).

Away from home

▸ Avoid distracting situations. (After one incident, I did my grocery shopping while she attended day care.)
▸ Make sure that your respite/day-care facility has an electronic system that alerts them if someone wanders.

Wandering, safe return

In spite of your best efforts, the unthinkable may happen—especially in the companionship or early dependent phases. During the independent phase, too much awareness exists. In the final phase, physical impairments abound.

▸ Join the Safe Return Program. Post the phone numbers of your local police department and Safe Return on your refrigerator.
▸ Take photos of your family member every year. Give copies to the local police (along with any other pertinent details) and keep several handy.
▸ Mentally practice describing her clothing of the day.

If it happens

▸ React quickly. (A family member can cover a great distance in a short time.)
▸ Call the local police and the Safe Return Program.
▸ Enlist others to help. Pass out pictures of your family member.

Project Lifesaver

One may live in the jurisdiction of one of the 250 police departments (in thirty-three states) that participate in this program. By using a one-ounce wrist transmitter (made by CareTrak), they have a 100% success rate so far of finding people who have wandered. CareTrak charges a monthly fee to maintain the equipment. To find out more about this program, visit their Web site at www.projectlifesaver.org. Interested police departments may call 757-546-5502.

Weight, maintaining

To understand fluctuations in weight better, one should record each weighing (including date) on a single piece of paper. (Also see Assumption #1 in Chapter 17.)

Losing weight

During the early phases of the disease, keeping a person's weight down may be a challenge. At one point, June's fingers became so fat that her wedding ring may have been causing pain. Overnight respite facilities asked me to remove the wedding ring. Taking a ring off a fat, swollen finger is difficult. Do it at the earliest opportunity.

Unlike some diet plans, the following simple ideas will work because they require no will power by a family member.

▸ Increase exercise for your family member.
▸ Reduce the quantity of items with fat. Substitute nonfattening snacks.
▸ Eliminate pastries and high cholesterol meat, switch to skim milk, and switch from ice cream to fat free frozen yogurt.
▸ Switch from butter/oleo to olive oil.
▸ Reduce carbohydrates and increase proteins.

Gaining weight

In the late phases, keeping weight up may be the challenge. In a nursing facility, June dropped to a low of 89 pounds. It took three months for her to gain twenty-one pounds and to look healthy again. Although I gradually backed off from this diet, she regained her normal weight of 135 pounds the following year. The following list of additional food helped:

▸ Buttered bread
▸ An afternoon snack of Carnation® Instant Breakfast using whole milk
▸ A large potato for dinner
▸ A large bowl of ice cream each night

Wheelchair (getting one into a car)

The following methods assume one has a compact car with a small trunk opening. Remove the foot rests from the wheelchair. Put it on its side and let gravity fold it (well-oiled hinges help).

Stronger caregiver

▸ Tilt the wheelchair so its front wheels rest on the rear bumper, almost into the car. Before lifting, keep your arms straight and knees bent and allow your back muscles to do the lifting. Keeping the front wheels on the bumper as a fulcrum, lift the rest of the wheelchair into the trunk. When removing, slide and balance the wheelchair on the outer back edge of the inside trunk. Then swing it down in a fluid motion.

Less strong (or injured) *caregiver*

▸ Get two pieces of scrap lumber (1" x 6" about five feet long) to use as ramps from the trunk to the ground. Prop them both on one side of the bumper, so tipping the wheelchair on its side after rolling it up the ramp will be easier. Space them apart to coincide with the spacing of the folded wheelchair wheels. Center the wheelchair's weight by tilting it onto its back wheels and get them unto the bottom of the boards. Step on the bottom of the boards to hold them securely in place and finish rolling the back wheels into the trunk. Turn the wheelchair sideways until both sets of wheels are in. Without lifting, get the rest of the wheelchair in by working it back and forth. (Don't forget to take the lumber along to get the wheelchair out of the trunk.)

Chapter 17
Good Examples of Bad Advice

During our seventeen-year journey with Alzheimer's disease, I often heard unkind, ineffective, inappropriate, or harmful advice and assumptions. This chapter encourages caregivers to be less accepting of what they hear or read.

BAD ADVICE #1: To reduce incontinence, withhold liquids after dinner.

This prevalent advice is solely for the convenience of the caregiver and ignores the needs of the sick person. It also violates a *secret of survival*—providing care with dignity. The practice may lead to constipation and dehydration. Once caregivers compromise one health issue, they may risk compromising others. From a practical point of view, changing a partially wet bed is no easier than changing a fully wet one.

BAD ADVICE #2: Caregivers should continue doing all the things that they have enjoyed.

Following this advice through year ten resulted in great frustrations. So I stopped doing almost everything that I did before, especially those things that I found tiring or difficult. Then I found new things to do that fitted my new life.

BAD ADVICE #3: Walk behind the person when helping to walk or climb stairs.

Except in the final few years, walking behind was far more difficult than leading.

BAD ADVICE #4: One should put a gate at the top of stairs to prevent wandering at night.

A strong or heavy Alzheimer's patient will probably crash through or fall over a gate. Putting a gate at the top of stairs may result in life-threatening injuries. Locking the door of the bedroom before going to bed is a safer, simpler, and less expensive solution.

Assumptions are a form of bad advice, but even worse because their perpetuation may cause some persons in the health care field to be dismissive of real problems. They did not prove accurate for my wife and may not be for your family member either.

ASSUMPTION #1: The disease is the primary cause of agitation, incontinence, stiffness, and weight loss.

Near sundown, articles frequently say that a person's agitation increases. My wife was too tired to become agitated at the end of a day. An exception occurred in a nursing home that consistently used physical restraints. Most studies have taken place in nursing homes. This behavior may be a result of the reduced size of the nursing home's second shift and consequent attempts to control patient behavior. In trying to understand agitation, I looked at it through June's eyes. In other words, what if one could not express fatigue, hunger, thirst, or other uncomfortable things? Babies cry. A person with Alzheimer's becomes agitated. Agitation had a real cause. It was simply up to the detective in me to find it.

At the end of the companionship phase, June started on drugs that caused incontinence immediately. When we stopped the drugs, incontinence stopped. After we restarted drugs the following year, incontinence restarted. When we later significantly reduced drugs, incontinence decreased significantly.

Stiffness did not start until June started on drugs. Her back formed a rigid arch, one arm looked as if it were in a cast, and her fingers had a claw like curl. After we significantly reduced certain drugs, these conditions stopped. Not until the middle of the final phase did this symptom reappear, when occasionally she did not immediately lower her head to her pillow at bedtime. Her hands, however, remained soft and pliable until she died.

During the first eighteen months on drugs, June lost twenty-six pounds before stabilizing for a year. After she stopped taking drugs, she regained her earlier weight loss. Then she went into a nursing facility for a long stay, where she lost twenty pounds. They tried to convince me that the disease caused the loss. After leaving that facility, however, she regained the weight lost there. As late as three months before she died, her weight remained at its normal level.

ASSUMPTION #2: One loses the ability to speak by the final stage.

At the end of the dependent phase, June amazed a home companion (who also worked at the day-care center) by the frequency of her speech at home. In addition, each year she added new words to her limited vocabulary. Because her speech was softer and less comprehensible by the middle of the final phase, one had to listen very closely.

ASSUMPTION #3: Grabbing is a sign of aggression.

The word *grabbing* has a very negative connotation. Others caring for your family member often use to justify isolation or physical and chemical restraints. A more appropriate word is clutching (as in *at straws*). Family members often desperately try to reach out for affection, reassurance, warmth, or physical support. The sick person may have suffered some loss in their fine motor control or simply forgotten how to touch nicely.

ASSUMPTION #4: Once one loses skills, one cannot regain them.

Believing this statement might discourage a caregiver from trying. (It discourages one enough that some things take a long time to accomplish.) My wife successfully relearned self-feeding, walking, climbing stairs, and using the toilet.

In the middle of the dependent phase, June spent lengthy stays in a nursing facility, a hospital, and a rehabilitation center. Once back at home, she relearned how to use both a spoon and a fork with minimum assistance.

After June's hip replacement, she could not follow the instructions that would have made her rehabilitation easier. With the aid of a walker and one person, however, she took her first hesitant steps after nine days. Five weeks later, she climbed her first few steps with assistance. Three months later, she walked alone. Five months after that, she climbed stairs with little assistance.

After three years, I wondered whether June could relearn toilet use. It took four months for her first success and more than a year for her to do so regularly. As late as her final year, she succeeded three-fourths of the time.

LESSONS LEARNED

By blindly following all *pied-piper* advice and assumptions, one will only create an atmosphere of hopelessness. By finding one's way past these challenges, however, one will gain confidence and inner strength. Moreover, one can gain the greatest need of a caregiver—hope.

Notes

Epilogue

Most caregivers care for their family members at home, even continuing past being recognized. Even if they might not love the person for whom they are caring, could caregivers do otherwise and come out of the experience a whole person? Could they ever again find happiness if they had not done their best for their family member? Thinking only from a selfish standpoint, one's mental and emotional survival should be an adequate reason to answer, "No."

However, more compelling reasons exist. Many people think that because persons with dementia do not always express feelings or thoughts, they do not have them. Close observation proves this assumption wrong. In some ways, persons with Alzheimer's are similar to a small child. They can express every emotion in some way. A new parent exults with each new occurrence in a baby's progress. A caregiver finds joy in every familiar word, gesture, or facial expression—perhaps a smile, a look of recognition, or an acknowledgment of some sort. With fewer joyful occasions as time passes, a caregiver takes even greater joy from them because of their rarity. Although those with dementia cannot fully talk, it is likely that each year, they will say words not spoken in the previous years of their illness. Except the last few days of life, they will give signs of awareness. That alone should make one want to continue to take care of them. Going through this experience, a caregiver can become a kinder, gentler, and more fully developed person.

We live in a fast-paced society, with less time for thoughtful reflection and healthy release of emotions. So it seems reasonable that most people will not think about caregiving. As our population ages, however, many will face this situation. Some will choose to step forward and care for their family members. One hopes that government assistance will become more oriented toward making it easier for them to do so at home.

One's background may make one ill prepared to be a caregiver. However, one will find that the personal qualities that one does have (e.g., spirituality, creativity, initiative, determination, and devotion to a family member) can compensate. As their family member deteriorates, caregivers will sometimes think that they cannot handle the next challenge. When the need arises, however, they can learn the required skills. This book should help others believe this, teach them how to get the needed skills, and shorten the time until they gain confidence in their abilities.

Appendix A
Music Videos

(Also see Video tapes/DVD in the Products chapter)

We only received only one television channel that played songs twenty-four hours a day—country music. These songs inspired me.

Alabama	*It Works*
Jessica Andrews	*I Will Be There for You*
Suzy Bogguss	*Letting Go*
Lisa Brokop	*How Do I Let Go*
Garth Brooks	*If Tomorrow Never Comes*
Garth Brooks	*The Dance*
Corbin and Hanner	*I Will Stand by You*
Dixie Chicks	*You Were Mine*
Diamond Rio	*You're Gone*
Patty Loveless	*How Can I Help You Say Goodbye*
Reba McEntire	*Is There Life Out There?*
Tim McGraw	*Can't Be Really Gone*
John Michael Montgomery	*I Swear*
Lorrie Morgan	*I Didn't Know My Own Strength*
Collin Raye	*Love, Me*
LeAnn Rimes	*You Light Up My Life*
Travis Tritt	*More Than You'll Ever Know*
Tanya Tucker	*Two Sparrows in a Hurricane*
Trisha Yearwood	*Where Your Road Leads*

The song, *Learning to Live Again*, from *The Chase*, a tape by Garth Brooks, became an audio favorite while driving.

GOLDEN OPPORTUNITY
Inspirational music videos (either tape or DVD) can be excellent gifts for a caregiver.

Appendix B
Activities of Daily Living

The National Association of Insurance Commissioners (NAIC) defined the six activities of daily living (ADL): bathing, dressing, eating, maintaining continence (control of bladder and bowel), toileting (mental ability to use the toilet), and transferring (physical ability to move oneself to another location).

In 1996, Congress passed the Kassebaum-Kennedy bill, naming the same six primary activities of daily living. It also defined a chronically ill person as needing assistance with at least two of these activities. Long-term care policies use these same definitions (See Insurance, private in the Financial chapter).

A caregiver must make many ADL tradeoffs. It may help others to see a sample ranking for the latter two phases of the disease.

▸ Maintaining continence helps to preserve the dignity of a family member and reduces urinary tract infections. It also raises the spirits of caregivers and makes their job easier.

▸ Eating continence-friendly food makes it possible to maintain continence.

▸ Moving from place to place helps to maintain regularity and overall health.

▸ Bathing enhances cleanliness, especially in case of incontinence.

▸ During the first two phases, dressing would be ranked higher because it raises the spirits of the ill person.

▸ The mental ability to use the toilet is last because a caregiver can compensate for the inability of the ill person.

Appendix C
Food recipes

Bean soup
Hurst sells a package of beans for ham flavored *15 Bean Soup*. The following recipe changes or additions appealed to me.
- ▸ To avoid accidentally getting a ham-hock bone, substitute smoked turkey sausage.
- ▸ Substitute Lite-salt in the water used to soak the beans.
- ▸ Add a heaping teaspoon of chili powder.
- ▸ Use a large can (28 oz.) of diced tomatoes.

Chili
Wick Fowler sells a *2-Alarm Chili Kit*. Buy two packages. The following recipe changes appealed to me.
- ▸ Substitute ground turkey breast.
- ▸ Use a large can (29 oz.) of tomato sauce and a large can (52 oz.) of red kidney beans.
- ▸ Add at least one teaspoon of plain cocoa powder.
- ▸ Use half the chili powder, half the salt, and omit the red pepper. Cooking it longer will bring out plenty of flavor.

Changes to both recipes
- ▸ Substitute bottled spring water.
- ▸ At least one large sweet onion adds flavor. (Putting it in the freezer for a short time before chopping should eliminate tears).
- ▸ Add at least one red pepper and clove of garlic, and a can (15 oz.) of whole kernel corn.

These recipes should make at least nine meals for two.
- ▸ Have plastic freezer containers available to freeze unused portions. Put one meal for two in each container.

Appendix D
Mental status tests

The mental status tests used to diagnose Alzheimer's were:

Bender Gestalt (thirty minutes)—it decided the accuracy of perception and detected brain damage.

Human Figure Drawings (thirty minutes)—they tested reasoning, spatial aptitude, and perceptual accuracy.

Minnesota Multiphasic Personality Inventory (one hour)—it measured emotional, motivational, and interpersonal and attitudinal characteristics, as distinguished from abilities.

Thematic Apperception Test (one hour)—it revealed habits of thought, attitudes, needs, and gave a composite picture of one's whole personality.

Wechsler Adult Intelligence Scale (Revised—one hour)—it estimated intelligence and classified some mental disorders.

Appendix E
Samples of NIH studies

Drugs

Guanfacine

Alzheimer's disease causes the loss of nerve cells that contain and use norepinephrine as their neurotransmitter. Guanfacine acts similarly to norepinephrine. This study tested the chemical's ability to improve memory and thinking.

Somatostatin

A chemical deficiency of a hormone called somatostatin is associated with Alzheimer's disease. A synthetic compound drug worked similarly to somatostatin. The study tested the benefits and safety of short-term treatment. The first study gave daily doses. A second study gave a continuous daily dose intravenously.

Tetrahydroaminoacridine (THA)

The brains of persons with Alzheimer's disease have severely diminished amounts of the neurotransmitter acetylcholine. THA increases acetylcholine levels. This study evaluated more rigorously the reported beneficial effect of THA. An initial screening included ten mental or physical examinations. The FDA ultimately approved this drug as Cognex (Tacrine Hydrochloride).

Research

The first inpatient stay involved mental status tests, which provided an objective record of her abilities. It also gave them a useful basis for comparison in the future. In addition, the staff gave laboratory tests including blood tests, brain scans, an ECG and EEG, a chest X-ray, and a spinal tap. A PET (Positron Emission Topography) scan measured the brain's breakdown of sugar, which provides the energy necessary for nerve cells to function properly. NIH is one of few locations in the United States able to do one.

Once a month for six months, she took half-day memory tests. A doctor also interviewed me, and then I completed various forms.

Some forms of the disease are hereditary. They could not, however, conclusively establish a link in our case.

Early in year five, June became an inpatient for two days. She had a spinal tap to learn the cerebrospinal fluid levels of various neurotransmitters (chemicals that help send electrical impulses in the brain). Later that year, she became an inpatient for four days for physician evaluations, mental status tests, and other laboratory tests.

At the beginning of the final phase, June participated in genetic testing regarding Apolipoprotein E (ApoE). ApoE is a plasma protein involved in cholesterol transport. Alzheimer's disease increases ApoE synthesis. Individuals have two copies of the gene for this protein, one inherited from each parent. Three different types of this gene exist. Researchers now think that one of those types (E4) is an important genetic susceptibility factor for Alzheimer's disease. If both parents passed down an E4 gene, an even higher risk exists. They drew one sample of blood to check on the gene and another sample for DNA extraction and storage. They planned to test it in the future as markers become available for defects in other genes. Since June's mother still lived, she agreed to provide information for this study. The doctor at NIA said it was a rare opportunity to look at two generations.

GOLDEN OPPORTUNITY

In the rush to the next scientific discovery, losing sight of the human equation may be easy for research scientists. They need to consider ways to help those who have helped them. For example, if they proved that the E4 gene had a connection to Alzheimer's, wouldn't it be appropriate to give gene information about the contributor to their family?

Appendix F
Emergency Medical Data

For _____(Blood type _____)
Who is a caregiver for _____
Who is normally at _____
▸ Call 911
▸ Take to _____Hospital
_____Road
      Exit _____ off the Capital Beltway
                         ( ) _____
▸ Dr. _____ ( ) _____
▸ Daughter _____ cell ( ) _____
                  office ( ) _____
                  home ( ) _____
▸ Mother-in-law _____ ( ) _____
▸ Son _____ cell ( ) _____
                  office ( ) _____
                  home ( ) _____
▸ Daughter-in-law _____ cell ( ) _____
                  office ( ) _____

LESSONS LEARNED

▸ Medical emergency instructions should be in large, bold type.

▸ Others caring for your family member should have a copy of the DNR and telephone numbers of companies that can repair utility problems. This includes air-conditioning and heating, cable TV, electricity, gas, plumbing, and water.

▸ One may live near several states and desire treatment outside one's home state. A 911 call results in going to the nearest medical facility for stabilization. One may then transfer to the hospital of your choice. In your emergency data, one should specify which ambulance service one wishes to do this.

Appendix G
Helpful care hints

Maintaining continence

Help in seating on the toilet four times a day (upon arising, mid AM, mid PM, and before bed). She needs about fifteen minutes each time with complete privacy. Give her water in a plastic glass each time. She can hold it herself. Use baby wipes.

Meals

Needs to eat a lot to keep up weight and strength. To avoid constipation, lots of grains, fruits, and vegetables are in the refrigerator. No sugar. Feed her with a spoon—no forks. If you place a glass or finger food in her hands, she can feed herself.

▸ Breakfast—Orange (peeled and sliced), bran cereal, toast with one tablespoon olive oil and jelly, banana

▸ Lunch—Soup, sandwich, fruit, milk

▸ Dinner—Turkey/bean soup is in a plastic container on top shelf of the refrigerator. A tuna casserole is also there. Add carrots, bread with olive oil, and vanilla frozen yogurt. On alternate nights, prepare an entree and a large salad with at least four raw vegetables. (Romaine lettuce, celery, broccoli, cauliflower, tomato, and red peppers are in the refrigerator.)

Baths

For full baths, seat her on the transfer bench in the tub. (She had a full bath/shampoo Sunday.) For sponge baths, only use water on her face. (Otherwise, chapping occurs.) Washcloths—Green for face, light blue for groin area. Flush that area daily with a hand-held shower (on *Gentle*)

Dressing

To prevent a blood blister on her left heel, keep shoes and socks on during the day.

** (The top strap of sandals should be strapped loosely.)

Exercise

Walk with her several times a day. She should **never** walk alone because she sits with nothing behind her.

Liquids

Give these additional liquids: water after brushing her teeth, cranberry juice twice daily, and milk daily. **No** ice (to avoid cracking a tooth).

Recreation

She watches music videos on CMT (Channel 111).

Morning

** The total morning routine takes about 2:30-3:00. To get her to day care early Monday, please plan accordingly.

Bedtime

June goes to bed at 8:00 PM and sleeps about ten hours on her back or right side. Raise the rails on both sides of the hospital bed. Keep a night-light on.

** Add an absorbent insert for the fitted brief.

Medicine

** Klonipin (0.25 mg)—AM and bedtime. After chewing, give water.

Questions

** You may reach me at _____ (My mobile phone number is _____).

** My daughter is at _____.

Day-care center: call _____ or _____ at _____.

** Addition or change since your last visit.

LESSONS LEARNED

For easy updating, these instructions should be broken into three parts:

▸ Data that changes little and applies to all providers of care.
▸ Additions that only pertain to home care providers.
▸ Additions that only pertain to the current season or a temporary medical condition.

Appendix H

Live-in agreement (sample)

I, _____(the home owner) agree to:

▸ Provide a basement apartment, storeroom, and utilities (electricity, gas, and water) at no charge.
▸ Pay for time more than sixty hours at the rate of $_____ per hour, and may provide money to eat dinner at inexpensive restaurants while caregiving.

I, _____(the home companion) agree to:

▸ Provide sixty hours of care a month.
▸ Make no changes or additions in the apartment, including the walls.
▸ Pay for damages.
▸ Not keep pets, have overnight guests, or provide care for others in this home.

Duties while providing care:
▸ Companionship and diversion from mischievous activities
▸ Preparation of simple meals and help while eating
▸ Guidance with dressing and undressing
▸ Assistance with bathing and dental hygiene (brushing and flossing)
▸ Supervision during use of the toilet

Other responsibilities:
▸ Maintain the area next to the basement outside entrance.

Either party, with thirty days written notice, may cancel this agreement.
This agreement is effective on _____

We both agree to the above.

_____   _____
Signature   Date   Signature   Date

Appendix I
Clothing Inventory

#	DESCRIPTION
____	BLOUSE
____	SHIRT
____	CULOTTES
____	SHORTS
____	SKIRTS
____	PANTS
____	UNDERCLOTHES
____	SOCKS
____	SHOES
____	SWEATER
____	SLIPPERS
____	NIGHT CLOTHES
____	ROBE
____	COAT
____	HAT
____	GLOVES
____	BRUSH
____	COMB
____	DEODORANT
____	DNR
____	INCONTINENCE SUPPLIES
____	MEDICINE
____	TOOTHBRUSH
____	TOOTHPASTE
____	VITAMINS
____	WASH BASIN KIT

Appendix J

Percent of respite cost

Phase/Live-ins Year		Day Care	Home Care	Nursing Home	Hospice
Ind 3	*				
Ind 4	*				
Ind 5	*				
Com 1	*				
Com 2	*	100			
Com 3	7	93	*		
Dep 1	15	56	11	18	
Dep 2		63	7	30	
Dep 3		34	1	65	
Dep 4		84		16	
Dep 5		80	2	18	
Fin 1		59		41	
Fin 2		69	2	29	
Fin 3		65	12	23	**
Fin 4		61		39	**
Aver	**2**	**64**	**4**	**30**	**

* A family member or friend provided care at no cost
** Medicare paid all of the cost

Appendix K
Vocabulary

Until the second year of the dependent phase (the year she started on drugs), June's speech was normal. In the middle of the last year of the dependent phase, we stopped the antipsychotic drug. She spoke more than twice as much the rest of that year.

In the middle of the next year (the first year of the final phase), we stopped the antianxiety drug. For the rest of that year, she spoke more than twice as much as she had the previous year.

Her speech peaked the next year. In her final year, she spoke about three times more than her first year on drugs. The total number of different words she spoke, however, decreased to only one-fourth of those in her peak year.

Longest sentences

Dependent 2—"Do you know what my mother said?" When I replied negatively, she said, "You're bad." A few moments later, "I was a bad girl. I'm sorry" (after a major incontinence accident).

Dependent 3—"Stay with me and let's play" (just before she got on the bus to day care).

Dependent 4—"Oh, how good. She loves it" (eating a Honeybell orange and cereal).

Dependent 5—"Oh, you're so nice" (after handing her a drink).

Final 1—"Isn't that cute" (while watching children on TV).

Final 2—"Oh, I don't know" (as I helped her get seated for dinner). She also spoke three amazingly long and intelligent sentences one night. In my amazement, I forgot to enter them in my journal. Later, I could not remember what she said (much like many of my dreams).

Final 3—"Wait a minute" (as I may have been going too fast in helping her into bed).

Final 4—"Thank you" (after I helped her into the car).

Appendix L
Maintaining skills

June could do the following things independently through these years:
Independent 2
> ‣ Hold jobs as a para-legal (her skill area)

Independent 3
> ‣ Travel by plane or Metro (subway)
> ‣ Hold a less demanding job
> ‣ Take classes (Weight Watchers and quilting)

Independent 5
> ‣ Spend time alone at home
> ‣ Do the laundry
> ‣ Help with the Christmas cards

Companionship 1
> ‣ Plant a flower garden
> ‣ Use revolving doors

Companionship 2
> ‣ Dress herself
> ‣ Travel abroad and entertain friends at home (with me)

Companionship 3
> ‣ Travel overnight by car (with me)
> ‣ Bathe
> ‣ Cut her food
> ‣ Sign our income-tax forms
> ‣ Cooperate with her ophthalmologist

Dependent 1
> ‣ Help herself to food from the refrigerator
> ‣ Eat out (with me)

Dependent 2
> ‣ Move from place to place alone
> ‣ Greet someone outside our family by name

June continued to do the following things, but only sporadically.
Dependent 3
> ‣ Respond to someone asking her name with her first or her birth name

Final 1
> ‣ Acknowledge good meals and my comments

Final 3
> ‣ Ask and answer questions
> ‣ Appraise a condition

Final 4
> ‣ Express pleasure/displeasure, agreement/disagreement, and needs
> ‣ Greet persons and acknowledge compliments or favors

Bibliography

BY A FAMILY MEMBER OR AN ILL PERSON

Alzheimer's disease

Bayley, John, *Elegy for Iris*, Saint Martin's Press, 1999.

Bayley, John, *Iris and Her Friends*, W. W. Norton, 2000. John was Iris Murdoch's husband. Producers told her story with the movie, *Iris*, starring Dame Judi Dench.

Brown, Dorothy S., *Handle With Care*, Prometheus Books, 1984. The author worked while caring for her mother. She had experience with live-in companions and nursing homes.

Burdick, Lydia, *The Sunshine on My Face*, Health Professionals Press, 2004.

Burdick, Lydia, and Jane Freeman, *Happy New Year to You!*, Health Professionals Press, 2006. One may share these latter two read-aloud books with someone with Alzheimer's.

Caldwell, Marianne, *Gone Without a Trace*, Elder Books, 1995. The author's mother disappeared and this book builds a good case for preventing wandering.

Davidson, Ann, *Alzheimer's, A Love Story: One Year in My Husband's Journey*, Carol Publishing, 1997. Ann was a primary caregiver for three years. The book covers incidents during one year.

Dyer, Joyce, *In a Tangled Wood: An Alzheimer's Journey*, SMU Press, 1996. This book covers observations of multiple patients during her mother's short stay inside an Alzheimer's unit.

Friel McGowin, Diana, *Living in the Labyrinth*, Delacorte, 1993. This autobiography is the author's chronicle of her battle with Alzheimer's Disease, the first from a patient's perspective.

Malachowski, Virginia, *Alzheimer's Disease*, Blisswood Books, 1987. The author compared her views of events with her mother's taped comments.

Marcell, Jacqueline, *Elder Rage*, Impressive Press, 2001. A very detailed account (sometimes humorous) of several years while the author mends her frail mother and turns her rebellious father around.

McAndrews, Lynn, *My Father Forgets*, Northern, 1990. This biography offers some insight into the devastation that Alzheimer's causes its victims and families. It has many recorded conversations.

Roach, Marion, *Another Name for Madness*, Houghton Mifflin, 1985. Besides her mother's biography through the first stage of the illness, the author tells about her emotions before placement in a nursing home.

Notes

Shanks, Lela Knox, *Your Name is Hughes Hannibal Shanks*, University of Nebraska Press, 1999. The author covers her philosophy and a biography of her husband.

Taylor, Richard, *Alzheimer's From the Inside Out*, Health Professionals Press, 2006. Diagnosed with Alzheimer's at age sixty-one, a former psychologist reveals something of his world.

Wall, Frank A., *Where Did Mary Go?*, Prometheus Books, 1996. This is a biography and pictorial essay about his wife. He also covers the seventeen lessons that he learned.

Womack, Dorothy, *Alzheimer's Angels: A Compilation of Poetry Honoring Caregivers and Victims of Alzheimer's Disease*, Writers Club Press, 2002. More than 200 poems by a fourteen-year caregiver.

Other senile dementia

Danforth, Art, *Living With Alzheimer's: Ruth's Story*, The Prestige Press, 1986. This biography covers Ruth's life and eventual death from Pick's Disease.

Doernberg, Myrna, *Stolen Mind: The Slow Disappearance of Ray Doernberg*, Algonquin Books of Chapel Hill, 1986. Myrna includes recorded conversations with her husband, who had Binswanger's Disease.

Other diseases

Caposella, Cappy, and Sheila Warnock, *Share the Care*, Simon & Schuster, 1995. This heart-warming book tells how a dozen friends divided responsibilities to care for a friend with cancer.

Cohen, Marion Deutsche, *Dirty Details*, Temple University Press, 1996. The author's husband had multiple sclerosis, and she tells about the years from his diagnosis until he went into a nursing facility.

Cooper, Joan Hunter, et al, *Fourteen Friends' Guide to Eldercaring*, 1999. Friends share personal anecdotes and solutions to situations faced in their caregiving experiences.

Horowitz, Karen E., *Witness to Illness*, Addison-Wesley, 1992. The author witnessed the deaths of her mother and grandmother from cancer. Then she kept a diary of her husband's battle with and recovery from cancer.

Martelli, Leonard J., William Messina, Fran D. Peltz, and Steven Petrow, *When Someone You Know Has AIDS*, Crown, 1993. They tell the story of ten couples and offer advice unique to this disease.

Starkman, Elaine M., *Learning to Sit in the Silence*, Papier-Mache Press, 1993. She and her husband took care of his mother for one year after a small stroke. This book covers the occurrences and the author's feelings.

SPECIALIZED BOOKS

Bell, Virginia, and David Troxel, *The Best Friend's Staff*, Health Professionals Press, 2001. They provide tools for training a healthcare staff.

Bell, Virginia, and David Troxel, *A Dignified Life*, HCI, 2002. This book provides a model for care built around effective communications and meaningful activities.

Boyer, Kim, and Mary Shapiro, *Alzheimer's and Dementia*, University of Nevada Press, 2006. This book is a practical legal guide for Nevada caregivers.

Fitzray, B. J., *Alzheimer's Activities: Hundreds of Activities for Men and Women with Alzheimer's Disease and Related Disorders*, Rayve Productions, 2001. The author outlines activities for daily and special occasions.

Heath, Angela, *Long Distance Caregiving*, American Source Books, 1993. This book covers nine major issues faced by long-distance caregivers, with recommendations for each issue.

Hodgson, Harriet W., *Alzheimer's: Finding the Words*, Chronimed, 1995. The book helps caregivers talk with persons that have Alzheimer's.

Nelson, James and Hilde, *Alzheimer's: Answers to Hard Questions for Families*, Doubleday, 1996. These bioethicists consider moral and ethical questions, such as conversations on life-prolonging procedures.

Oliver, Rose and Frances Bock, *Coping with Alzheimer's: A Caregiver's Emotional Survival Guide*, Dodd Mead, 1989. Using Rational Emotional Therapy, the authors describe more than a half dozen emotions.

Pollen, Daniel A., *Hannah's Heirs*, OUP, 1993. Most of this book covers genetics, but also includes the history of several generations of one family.

Sheridan, Carmel, *Failure Free Activities for the Alzheimer's Patient*, Dell, 1987. It covers crafts, exercise, food, games, gardening, music, reminiscence, and solo activities.

Warner, Mark L., *The Complete Guide to Alzheimer's-Proofing Your Home*, Purdue University Press, 1998. This guide covers how to renovate or redecorate one's home for the disabled.

Notes

FOR CHILDREN

Bahr, Mary, *The Memory Box*, Albert Whitman, 1992. When Gramps realizes he has Alzheimer's disease, he starts a memory box with his grandson to keep memories of all the times they have shared.

Gold, Susan Dudley, *Alzheimer's Disease*, Crestwood House, 1996. Using a biography of her father, the author discusses the causes, effects, and treatments.

Kroll, Virginia, *Fireflies, Peach Pies, & Lullabies*, Simon & Schuster, 1995, age 5-9. Francie helps others remember her great-granny Annabel rather than the shell she became as Alzheimer's ran its course.

Shecter, Ben, *Great-Uncle Alfred Forgets*, Harper Collins, 1996. A great-niece takes Alfred, who has Alzheimer's disease, for a walk and gently and patiently answers all his seemingly absurd questions.

FOR YOUNG ADULTS

Derby, Pat, *Visiting Miss Pierce*, Farrar-Straus-Giroux, 1986. Barry gets a school assignment to visit an elderly woman in the early stage of senile dementia. Over the weeks, Barry learns about her and himself.

GENERAL ALZHEIMER'S BOOKS

Carter, Rosalynn, *Helping Yourself Help Others,* Random House, 1994. The purpose of this book is to encourage, empathize, and advocate. It also quotes caregivers upset about the current information available.

Cohen, Donna, and Carl Eisdorfer, *The Loss of Self,* WW Norton, 2001-revised edition. These two health care managers cover about a dozen issues, with 134 pages devoted to causes and diagnosis of the disease.

Coughlan, Patricia B., *Facing Alzheimer's*, Ballantine, 1993. Eight women, who lived through their husbands' declines, talk about how they faced the decisions they had to make.

Cutler, Neal and John Sramek, *Understanding Alzheimer's Disease*, University Press of Mississippi, 1996. These two health care managers focus primarily on research, causes and diagnosis.

Fish, Sharon, *Alzheimer's*, Shaw, 1996. It includes causes, symptoms, treatment, handling emotions, and resources. One chapter covers whether one should use a nursing home.

Gillick, Muriel R., *Tangled Minds*, Dutton, 1998. This candid doctor tells how she made decisions regarding a composite woman from her diagnosis to death.

Gruetzner, Howard, *Alzheimer's*, Wiley, 2001-revised edition. The author emphasizes research, symptoms, phases, understanding behavior, and depression within both the caregiver and the family member.

Hay, Jennifer, *Alzheimer's and Dementia*, Peoples Medical Society, 1996. Research on causes, defines the many types of dementia, tells where caregivers can find help, and answers common questions.

Heston, Leonard and June A. White, *The Vanishing Mind*, W H Freeman, 1995. This book has unique scientifically compiled charts on longevity and percentages of misdiagnoses.

Hodgkinson, Liz, *Alzheimer's Disease*, Ward Lock (UK), 1996. This overview includes resources within Great Britain.

Kindig, Mary Norton, and Molly Carnes, *Coping with Alzheimer's Disease and Other Dementing Illnesses*, Singular, 1993. It gives information about senile dementia, finding assistance, and making plans.

Mace, Nancy, and Peter Rabins, *The 36-Hour Day*, Johns Hopkins University, 2006-revised edition. This book includes many definitions and covers diagnosis, causes, research, and nursing facility placement.

Markin, R. E., *The Alzheimer's Cope Book*, Citadel, 1992. The author designed this book for recently diagnosed persons. It also covers scientific progress.

Mathiasen, Patrick, *An Ocean of Time*, Scribners, 1997. This psychiatrist tells anecdotes in the lives of thirteen of his patients.

Post, Stephen G., *The Moral Challenge of Alzheimer Disease*, Johns Hopkins, 1995. The author philosophically discusses dementia, including respect, ethics, one's right to comfort, assisted-suicide, and euthanasia.

Powell, Lenore S., and Kate Courtice, *Alzheimer's Disease: A Guide for Families and Caregivers*, Addison-Wesley, 2002-revised edition. It emphasizes the emotional side of Alzheimer's, diagnosis, and research.

Reisberg, Barry, *A Guide to Alzheimer's Disease*, The Free Press, 1981. The book includes origins, evolution, medical treatment, and future directions.

Wolf-Klein, Gisele P., and Arnold P. Levy, *Keys to Understanding Alzheimer's Disease*, Barron, 1992. It covers definitions, treatments, and what to tell children, grandchildren, friends, and colleagues.

Memory, Johns Hopkins White Papers # 015057, 2005. This paper discusses protecting one's memory as one gets older.

DRUGS

The Pill Book, Bantam Books, 1996. This book helps to understand reactions to various drugs. Some supermarkets sell it. If this book and the pharmacy have differences, check with your doctor.

Index

Symbols

911 85, 141, 187

A

A.M. Best 44
AAA 30, 172
AARP 9, 45, 49, 50, 108, 158
Ability to speak 178
Accounting worksheet 67
Activities of daily living 31, 32, 34,
    35, 37, 44, 83, 94, 135, 182
Adduction pillow 77
Adenna 76
Advance Medical Directive 48
Advice to others who provide care
    156
After a hip replacement 77, 78,
    144, 159
Agitation 37, 63, 151, 177
Air mattress 58, 77, 150
Alabama 181
Alzheimer's Association 107
Alzheimer's Disease Education &
    Referral Center 107
Alzheimer's Disease International
    113
Alzheimer's unit 92
Ambidexterity 18
Andrews, Jessica 17, 181
American Bar Association 49
American Health Assistance Founda-
    tion 108
American Society of Consultant
    Pharmacists 68
Anger 16
Antianxiety drugs 56, 63, 64
Anticipation 24
Antidepressants 63
Antipsychotic drugs 63
Anxiety 31, 35
ApoE 186
Appetite 34, 127
Area Agency on Aging 42, 96, 104,
    107, 109, 110, 111
Assessing care 98

Assets 40, 42, 47, 48, 50
Assumptions 176, 177, 179
Automobile 137
Autopsy 60
Awareness 30, 33, 35, 36, 37, 61,
    64, 155, 156, 172, 180

B

Baby monitors 85
Bad Advice 176
Balance 26, 72, 136, 152
Balancing caregiving with caring for
    yourself 33
Bath transfer bench 25, 116, 133
Bathtub mat 70, 117
Bathtub non-slip strips 85
Bedroom 149, 169
Bedroom/dressing area 169
Bedsores 58
Bedtime 150, 189
Bender Gestalt 184
Bibs 71
Blair 81
Blood pressure monitor 71
Blood/toxin tests 55
Blow dryer 35, 71, 119
Blue Ridge Parkway 165
Body language 156
Bogguss, Suzy 181
Brokop, Lisa 181
Brooks, Garth 181

C

Calendar 152
Caller ID 84
Car 29, 32, 138, 147, 158
Care hints 188
Care rules 20
Carpenter, Mary Chapin 37
Certificate of Medical Necessity
    43, 74
Certified nursing aides 88
Changing area 134
Chewable pills 65, 66
Children of Aging Parents 108
Church 17, 106

Churchill, Winston 18, 119
Clothes 18, 31, 32, 69, 70, 71,
    121, 122, 149, 150, 151,
    154, 158, 163, 169
Clothing Inventory 191
Clutching 117, 123, 151, 152
Cognex 185
Communications 153
Companion 15, 33, 89, 141,
    178, 190
Companionship Phase 19, 20, 30,
    51, 56, 63, 64, 87, 116, 121,
    126, 165
Compliments 154, 157, 194
Constipation 64, 100
Constipation, easing 157
Consumer Product Safety Commis-
    sion 171
Consumer Reports 96
Continence-friendly food
    130, 134, 182
Cooking 32, 90, 105, 165, 132,
    170, 183
Corbin and Hanner 17, 181
Cord shorteners 169
Corinthians 17
Cornerstones 19, 20, 23, 25
Cost Control 66
Cranberry juice 59, 189
CT Scan 55
Culottes 73
Cups, spill-proof 73

D

Day care transportation 25, 103,
    111, 152
Day-care 19, 22, 30, 31, 33-38, 49,
    69, 74, 76, 88, 90, 103, 109,
    157, 159, 162, 163, 165-167,
    173, 178, 189
Dead bolts 36, 73, 172
Death Benefit 47
Decrease in appetite 127
Dependent Phase 21, 23-26, 33, 51,
    52, 56, 60, 63, 64, 71, 72,
    74, 88, 91, 116, 121, 126,
    128, 133, 135, 139, 141-143,
    145, 153, 154, 159, 162,
    164-167, 178, 193
Depression 55, 60, 110, 198

Desert Rhapsody 24, 85, 86
Diagnosis 28, 29, 40, 48, 50,
    55, 56, 108-110, 196, 198, 199
Diamond Rio 181
Disability Benefit 46
Dixie Chicks 181
DNR 62, 89, 187
Dog 32
Double meanings 155
Dr. Leonard's 81, 196, 199
Draw-sheet 76
Driving, stopping 157
Drug prescription and monitoring 56
Drug trials 30, 59, 61, 67
Drugs 6, 9, 20, 23, 35-38, 56,
    60, 61, 63, 64, 66, 67,
    97, 111, 115, 127, 128, 134,
    143, 160, 163, 177, 185, 199
Durable medical equipment 43, 45
Durable Power of Attorney
    48, 49, 97
DVD 84-86, 181

E

Early onset 9, 40, 55, 87
Early onset income 40
Egg-crate pad 58, 75
Elder Care Locator 95, 100, 109
Electric Toothbrush 52
Electrical 169
Electroencephalogram (EEG) 55
Emergency information 159, 171
Emergency Medical Data 159, 187
Emergency signalers 73, 105
en Como Agua Para Chocolate 20
Ethical Society 111
Exercise 90, 91, 100, 127, 141,
    150, 159, 167, 174, 188, 197
Expense records 41

F

Faith in Action 109
Falling Risk Assessment 160
Falls, preventing 160
Family, immediate 109
Fatigue 16, 150, 177
Faulkner, William 17
FDA 61, 66, 67, 185
Federal Trade Commission 74
Feeding 39, 61, 74, 100, 101, 127,
    128, 153

Notes

Feet and nail care 161
Final Phase 21, 37, 52, 116,
    126, 143, 144, 146, 164
Final phase 106, 115, 122, 128,
    137, 139, 142-145, 153-155
Fire 96, 170
First Aid 58, 80, 167
Flexibility 24
Flying 172
Food buying 130
Food preparation 132
Food recipes 183
Foreign Student Service Council 88
Francis, Dick 165
FreeCell 18
Friends of Disabled Adults and
    Children 86
Frustration 17, 19

G

Genetic testing 186
Geriatric chair 37, 43, 52, 74, 83,
    86, 130, 133, 136, 138, 139,
    160, 161, 163, 166
Getting into the tub 138
Getting on the bus 143
Getting up from furniture 141
Getting up from the floor 141
Gloves 52, 72, 81, 135
Gloves, disposable 76
Going to bed 139, 177
Government assistance 180
Grab bars 69, 169
Graham Field 70
Guanfacine 185
Guilt 16, 20

H

Haband 81
Hair appointments 162
Haley, Alex 154
HALT 49
Hand-held foods 126, 128
Hand-held shower 25, 59, 116,
    117, 188
HDIS 81
Heel boot 75, 161

Hiding items 152
Highest allowable dose 67
Hip protectors 85
Hip replacement 23, 36, 57, 61,
    75, 93, 133, 138, 144, 165
Hopelessness 179
Hospice 38, 48, 77, 103
Hospital and Healthcare Association
    48
Hospital bed 43, 75, 78, 86, 119,
    150, 189
Hospitalization 44, 57
Hours of care 166, 190
How Green Was My Valley 25
Human Figure Drawings 184

I

I Will Be There for You 17, 181
Identification bracelet 35, 111, 150
Immediate cause of death 62
Inadequacy 22
Income tax 42, 47
Incontinence brief insert 76
Incontinence briefs 75
Increasing communication 153
Independent Phase 27, 51, 60, 87,
    109, 163, 165, 173
Interdental Brush 52, 53
Internet 46, 47, 70, 71, 76, 80,
    83, 110
Invacare 81
IRS 42, 89
Isolation 23, 178

J

Jackets 72, 172
Judgment 29, 30, 152

K

Kassebaum-Kennedy bill 182
Kitchen 162, 170
Klonipin 64, 189

L

Labor-contract for caregivers 15
Laboratory tests 185
Laughter 26, 64, 133, 157
Lawyer 49
Leg separator 58, 77

Letter 22, 30, 47, 49, 59, 64, 66, 67
Lift 39
Light switches 74, 170
Liquid medicines 66
Liquids 163, 189
Live-in agreement 88
Live-ins 88, 192
Living will 48, 49, 97
Loan-closet 86
Lodgings 172
Long-distance caregiving 46, 73, 105, 109, 109
Long-term care 9, 44, 45, 102, 105, 108, 110, 112, 182
Loss of appetite 64
Loss of awareness 64
Loss of libido 64
Loveless, Patty 181

M

Maintaining continence 59, 100, 134, 182, 188
Maintaining skills 100
Manage time better 22
Mattress, air 77
Mayo Clinic 55
McEntire, Reba 181
McGraw, Tim 181
Medicaid 10, 42, 47
Medical Letter 67
Medical Records 57
Medicare 40, 42-44, 58, 74, 75, 77, 82, 83, 92, 96, 104
Mental Status Tests 55, 184, 185
Minnesota Multiphasic Personality Inventory 184
Moban (Molindone) 63, 67
Montgomery, John Michael 181
Morgan, Lorrie 181
Move from place to place 35
MRI 60
Music 17, 34, 85, 97, 127, 133, 151, 166, 181, 189, 197
Music Videos 17, 24, 97, 133, 181

N

National Academy of Elder Law Attorneys 49

National Association of Insurance Commissioners 45, 182
National Hospice and Palliative Care 48, 104
National Institute of Mental Health (NIMH) 60
National Institute of Neurological Disorders and Strokes 60
National Institute on Aging 60, 107, 111
National Institutes of Health 26, 28, 59
National Library of Medicine 67
Neuro-psychiatrist 28, 30, 35, 55, 56, 94, 109
Neurologist 55
Nightgowns 72
NIH studies 185
Non-latex rubber gloves 52
Nursing facilities 21, 72, 76, 91
Nursing facility care 98
Nursing facility costs 100
Nursing facility experiences 92
Nursing facility, finding a good one 95
Nursing facility, preparing to enter 97
Nursing facility types 92
Nursing home 43, 69, 92, 95, 96, 104, 105, 177, 192, 195
Nursing Home Compare 96
Nursing Home Reform Law 95

O

Ombudsman 105, 108, 110
Operative report 57
Ophthalmologist 58, 194
Orthopedic surgeon 56

P

Pants 72, 73, 122, 123
Pastimes 18
Personal Emergency Response System 74
PET scan 60, 185
Pet 32, 33
Pharmacy 66, 79, 101, 199
Philosophy on dying 39
Photo 33
Physical coordination 29
Pill Book 67, 199

Notes

Pill organizers 77
Placement of dishes and utensils 127
Plastic covering 78
Podiatrist 56, 161
Poison Control Center 53, 81, 171
Power of Attorney 46, 48
Prayer 25
Primary care physician 56
Project Lifesaver 173
Projects 22, 23, 90
Prompts 66, 128, 139
Psychologist 55

Q

Quiet time 22, 24, 165

R

Rashes 75, 119
Raye, Collin 181
Reaching out 23
Recipes 20, 183
Recreation 165, 189
Red Cross 58
Regaining skills 171
Relaxation 19, 101, 150
Religion 110
Repetitive questions 151
Respite care summary 101
Respite cost 102, 192
Retirement 30, 40, 41, 46, 47
Retirement Benefits 40, 46, 47
Rimes, LeAnn 181
Roosevelt, Theodore 17
Routines 17, 132, 166, 168
Runner, plastic 78

S

Safe Return Program 111, 173
Safety 35, 78, 82, 122, 168
Safety support vest 78, 147, 160, 165
Sammons 70, 75, 76
Scooting 82, 152
Sedation 54
Seizure 104
Self-feeding 127, 128, 129, 132, 178
Senior Care Pharmacist 68
Sense of accomplishment 22

Shoes 72, 81, 94, 123, 160, 188
Short-term memory loss 28
Shorts 73
Showers 116
Simplify 20
Skilled nursing units 92
Skills, maintaining 171
Skills, regained 134
Social Security 29, 40-42, 46, 47, 89
Socks 72, 73, 123, 149
Somatostatin 185
Something to look forward to 21
Speech 63, 153, 171, 178
Spinal tap 185
Spirituality 15, 25, 39, 180
Spoon, measuring 79
Stair lift 39, 79, 119, 144, 145
Stairs (down only) 142
Stairs (up only) 143
Standard & Poor's 44
State Social Services Department 111
Stiffness 64, 177
Stimulating/preventing action 155
Stress 17, 19, 24, 127
Stretching 24, 159, 160
Sundown 177
Support group 23, 33, 54, 69, 88, 111

T

T. Rowe Price 48
Talk to Her 156
Teeth care 51
Telephone answering machine 84
Telephone, cordless 85
Telephone, mobile 84
Tetrahydroaminoacridine (THA) 185
Thematic Apperception Test 184
Thermal glove liners 72
Thermometers 82
Things I least enjoy 25
Thoreau, Henry 17
Toilet safety frame 82, 134
Toilet seat cover 82
Transfer (gait) belt 82
Transfer bench 70, 116, 133, 138, 188
Travel 171

Notes

Notes

Tremors 38, 64
Tritt, Travis 181
Trust 40, 46, 48, 50
Tucker, Tanya 181

U

U.S. Department of Veterans Affairs 112
U.S. Senate Special Committee on Aging 106
Uncontrolled movements 37, 63
Underpads 77, 149
Undershirts 73, 149
Urinary tract infection 59, 83, 94, 127
Urine specimen collection bowl 83
USAA 159

V

VCR 84, 97
Videotapes 84, 85
Visiting Nurses Association 58
Visualization 26
Vocabulary 153, 171, 178, 193

W

Walkers 83
Walking 16, 145
Wandering 172, 173
Wandering, preventing 172
Wandering, safe return 173
Washington & Old Dominion bike trail 165
WebMD 55
Wechsler Adult Intelligence Scale 184
Weekly Minder 28, 29
Weight loss 94, 150, 177
Weight, maintaining 174
Wellness Letter 49, 59
Wheelchair 36, 43, 74, 78, 82, 83, 103, 136, 147, 148, 174, 175
White House 165
Wills 48, 49, 50
Window locks 84, 173
Wintergreen Mountain 23

X

X-rays 55, 57

Y

Yearwood, Trisha 181

How to order additional copies of this book

(Make a copy of this page and
give it to a friend in need or members of your support group)

Please send a copy of *Alzheimer's Care with Dignity* to:

_____
Name

_____
Address

_____
City   State   Zip code

_____
E-mail address (optional)

Please send me ___ copy[s] of *Alzheimer's Care with Dignity*.
I have enclosed $24.95 [U.S. Dollars] per book[s].

(VA residents: Add 5% sales tax for a total of $26.20)

Shipping: Free for all Limited First Editions.
(Normally ships USPS media mail within one business day)

Make check payable to Care with Dignity and mail to:

Care with Dignity
P.O. Box 861646
Warrenton, VA 20187

For credit card orders, go to
www.dementiacaregiving.com
E-mail questions to
carewithdignity@earthlink.net